MARKUS HAUN
Kapellenweg 16
D-69121 Heidelberg
markus.haun@posteo.de

Psychiatric Diagnosis Revisited

Stijn Vanheule

Psychiatric Diagnosis Revisited

From DSM to Clinical Case Formulation

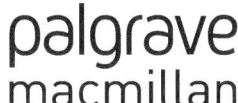

Stijn Vanheule
Ghent University
Ghent, Belgium

ISBN 978-3-319-44668-4   ISBN 978-3-319-44669-1   (eBook)
DOI 10.1007/978-3-319-44669-1

Library of Congress Control Number: 2017930174

© The Editor(s) (if applicable) and The Author(s) 2017
This book was advertised with a copyright holder in the name of the publisher in error, whereas the author holds the copyright.
This work is subject to copyright. All rights are solely and exclusively licensed by the Publisher, whether the whole or part of the material is concerned, specifically the rights of translation, reprinting, reuse of illustrations, recitation, broadcasting, reproduction on microfilms or in any other physical way, and transmission or information storage and retrieval, electronic adaptation, computer software, or by similar or dissimilar methodology now known or hereafter developed.
The use of general descriptive names, registered names, trademarks, service marks, etc. in this publication does not imply, even in the absence of a specific statement, that such names are exempt from the relevant protective laws and regulations and therefore free for general use.
The publisher, the authors and the editors are safe to assume that the advice and information in this book are believed to be true and accurate at the date of publication. Neither the publisher nor the authors or the editors give a warranty, express or implied, with respect to the material contained herein or for any errors or omissions that may have been made. The publisher remains neutral with regard to jurisdictional claims in published maps and institutional affiliations.

Cover illustration: Michaël Borremans, "The Egg IV", 2012, 42,0 x 36,0 cm, oil on canvas, photographer: Peter Cox, courtesy Zeno X Gallery, Antwerp

Printed on acid-free paper

This Palgrave Macmillan imprint is published by Springer Nature
The registered company is Springer International Publishing AG
The registered company address is: Gewerbestrasse 11, 6330 Cham, Switzerland

Other books by Stijn Vanheule:
The Subject of Psychosis—A Lacanian Perspective (Palgrave Macmillan, 2011).
Diagnosis and the DSM—A Critical Review (Palgrave Macmillan, 2014)

Acknowledgments

Many people supported me while researching and writing this book. My collaborators at the Department of Psychoanalysis and Clinical Consulting at Ghent University provided me with support and inspiration, for which I am grateful. The same is true for the many colleagues that I regularly meet and have met in the clinical setting, and for the experts by experience including Brenda Froyen, Ingrid Lammerant, and Hind Fraïhi, who, with their personal stories, inspired me to refine my ideas. Special thanks to Ignaas Devisch, with whom I discussed several key ideas that are discussed in Chap. 4. Above all I want to thank the psychology students following my classes on Clinical Psychological Assessment at Ghent University between 2006 and 2016. Their presence, curiosity, and concerns invited me to articulate my ideas as clearly as possible. Finally I am most grateful to Clare Murphy. She not only copy-edited the manuscript but also joined me in my lines of reasoning, thus pointing to ideas that needed further clarification.

Contents

1	**Introduction**	1
	Other References	6
2	**Dynamics of Decision-Making: The Issue of Reliability in Diagnosis**	7
	Diagnosis and the DSM	7
	From Prototype to Checklist: A Brief History	8
	Commotion in Psychiatry, Part I: Diagnosis Under Fire in the 1970s	16
	Commotion in Psychiatry, Part II: Critical Researchers Dethrone the Psychiatric Ethos	28
	Commotion in Psychiatry, Part III: Deinstitutionalization, Rationalization, Medicalization, and Fuzzy Decision-Making	40
	Neo-Kraepelinian Restoration	44
	Diagnostic Reliability Since the DSM-III	52
	Conclusion	67
	Other References	70
3	**Symptom and Context: The Issue of Validity in Diagnosis**	79
	Toward a Functional Account of Psychopathology	79

How the DSM Takes into Account Context	80
The Paradox of Polythetic Descriptive Diagnosis	84
Sign-Based Diagnosis	87
Beyond Sign-Based Diagnosis: Symptoms as Personal Constructions	90
Intermezzo: Lacan's Position	101
The Search for Biomedical Referents	105
Toward an Era of Biopsychopathology?	110
The Mental Disorder: What Kind of Kind?	119
Conclusion	125
Other References	126

4 From Mental Suffering to Mental Disorder and Back Again — 133

What Do We Diagnose?	133
Psychopathology	136
Psychopathology Versus Abnormality	138
What Is Pathos?	144
A Plea for Studying the Quality and Circumstances of Mental Suffering	150
DSM-5: A Matter of Disorders	153
What About Suffering: *Verstehen* or *Gardez-vous de comprendre*?	158
Conclusion	161
Other References	163

5 Working with Clinical Case Formulations: Methodological Considerations — 167

Mapping Mental Health Problems	167
Function-Oriented Diagnosis	169
Case Construction	172
Qualitative Research as a Methodological Framework	174
Quality Assurance in Diagnostic Case Formulation	179
Reflexivity	180

Reflexivity in the Context of Function-Oriented Case
    Formulation   184
Aiming at Validity and Reliability: A Matter of Careful
    Verification   193
Reliability Considered Closely   197
A Closer Look at Validity   200
Conclusion   205
Other References   207

Bibliography   213

Other References   214

Index   233

List of Figures

Fig. 3.1	Triangular model of symptom formation	101
Fig. 4.1	Two orthogonal axes on which Ricoeur situates mental suffering	146

List of Tables

Table 2.1	Overview of three sets of norms for evaluating the kappa statistic	24
Table 2.2	Kappa coefficients for DSM-II categories, adapted from Spitzer and Fleiss (1974, p. 344), and three sets of interpretations of the Kappa coefficient using different norms	25
Table 2.3	Kappa coefficients for research diagnostic criteria disorders adapted from Spitzer et al. (1978, p. 779), and three sets of interpretations of the kappa coefficient using different norms	49
Table 2.4	Kappa coefficients from the DSM-III field trials, adapted from Spitzer et al. (1979), and three sets of interpretations of the kappa coefficient using different norms	53
Table 2.5	Kappa coefficients from SCID-I test-retest study in psychiatric patients by Williams et al. (1992), and three sets of interpretations of the kappa coefficient using different norms	56
Table 2.6	Kappa coefficients from SCID-I test-retest study in non-patients by Williams et al. (1992), and three sets of interpretations of the kappa coefficient using different norms	57

Table 2.7	Kappa coefficients from SCID-II test-retest study in psychiatric patients by First et al. (1995), and three sets of interpretations of the kappa coefficient using different norms	58
Table 2.8	Kappa coefficients from SCID-II test-retest study in non-patients by First et al. (1995), and three sets of interpretations of the kappa coefficient using different norms	58
Table 2.9	Kappa coefficients from the DSM-5 field trials in adult patients (Regier et al. 2013) and three sets of interpretations of the kappa coefficient using different norms	60
Table 2.10	Kappa coefficients from the DSM-5 field trials in pediatric patients (Regier et al. 2013) and three sets of interpretations of the kappa coefficient using different norms	61
Table 2.11	Kappa coefficients from SCID test-retest study in psychiatric patients by Chmielewski et al. (2015), and three sets of interpretations of the kappa coefficient using different norms	65
Table 2.12	Kappa coefficients from audio-recording reliability study in psychiatric patients by Chmielewski et al. (2015), and three sets of interpretations of the kappa coefficient using different norms	66

1

Introduction

Worldwide an increasing number of people suffer from mental health problems. In 1990 a study on the global burden of disease attributable to mental or substance use disorders estimated that they accounted for more than a quarter of all non-fatal diseases. Between 1990 and 2010 the burden of psychiatric disorders further increased by 37.6% (Whiteford et al. 2013). This observation brought the World Health Organization to formulate a global action plan that aims to fight mental distress and disability, and to promote mental health (World Health Organization 2013).

At the same time numerous scholars have been increasingly warning us against the tendency toward overdiagnosis. More and more, common suffering and the discontents of daily life are being framed as diseases, even in the absence of severe impairment, which undermines the self-reliance of people dealing with such issues (Bolton 2013). A good illustration of this can be found in the work of Allen Frances (2013). Frances chaired the task force that prepared the previous version of the *Diagnostic and Statistical Manual of Mental Disorders* (DSM) of the American Psychiatric Association, which is a widely used instrument for diagnosing psychiatric disorders. One key message he now conveys is that under the influence of diverse stakeholders, like medical associations and the pharmaceutical industry, the stresses and sorrows of ordinary life are being increasingly medicalized. This wrongly stigmatizes people and inauspiciously encourages medical consumption.

These messages provide us with a paradox: on the one hand the burden of mental distress is serious, yet, on the other hand a substantial amount of diagnoses seem to be trivial. This paradox cannot be neglected, and points to the heart of all mental health-related professional action: diagnoses should accurately grasp the problems people suffer from, and should not be influenced by the whims and fancies of third parties that might profit at the expense of potential patients. Indeed, the diagnoses that professionals give should be valid and reliable, such that adequate action can be taken. Yet, what kind of diagnosis should guide further action? And what criteria should we take into account when assessing the value and impact of our diagnoses? These questions are central to this book. My research has brought me to think critically about classificatory diagnosis and to appreciate clinical case formulations.

In 2013 the American Psychiatric Association published the fifth version of the *Diagnostic and Statistical Manual of Mental Disorders* (DSM-5). For many academics and clinicians the DSM has a scientific credibility that it does not deserve. Numerous people believe that the manual provides a common language that enhances straightforward communication about mental health problems, and are convinced that the disorders described in the DSM comprise objective realities. These convictions are naïve and mistaken.

In popular press, the DSM is frequently coined as "the bible of psychiatry" and this is precisely how the handbook seems to function: people *believe* in its accuracy and legitimacy, largely without question. The manual could also be said to function somewhat at the base of the economy of psychiatry. Not only does it facilitate a belief system, but also survives as an important economic device for managing the flow of money invested into mental health care. It is on the basis of this classificatory system that decisions are made on issues such as the reimbursement of treatments, the right to financial aid, and the allocation of means across health care providers.

With this book I argue that the value of the DSM-5, and previous versions of the handbook, should not be taken for granted: the manual should be closely assessed and discussed. End users of the DSM-5 should not assume that the handbook is "good" or "useful," but become cognizant of its strengths and weaknesses, including its theoretical underpinnings and its position in historical debates on the scientific status of psychiatry and clinical psychology. Two chapters of this book discuss the reliability and validity of the DSM. Starting from a critique of the limitations that are inherent to classificatory diagnosis I subsequently discuss what I consider as a better alternative: *clinical case constructions that provide a detailed account of people's symptoms and functioning, and do not neglect the dimension of the subject.* Clinical case construction allows contextualized and personalized diagnosis. On the condition that the quality of such a narrative approach to diagnosis is optimized, working with clinical case constructions enables a more valid and reliable approach to mental health problems.

Chapter 2 focuses on the reliability of the DSM-5 and previous versions of the handbook. In the early days of psychiatry, diagnosis did not begin from checklists of symptoms, but from elaborate prototypical descriptions of a diverse range of psychopathology. Guided by administrative purposes these descriptions gave rise to classification systems such as the DSM. An important impetus for the switch to checklist-based diagnosis can be found in harsh discussions on the fundaments and the practice of psychiatry during the 1960s and 1970s. In these years, psychiatry was in crisis: several academic researchers demonstrated that psychiatric diagnosis was unreliable, critical scholars pointed to weak points in the overall ethos of psychiatry, and societal changes challenged the practice of psychiatry. A group of so-called neo-Kraepelinian psychiatrists responded to the malaise in the discipline by defining psychiatry as a strictly medical discipline and thus replacing the method of diagnosis with a criteria-based system. Checklist-based diagnosis is often believed to be more scientifically sound than narrative-based diagnosis. However, in this chapter I demonstrate that this is not the case: DSM-5 diagnosis is by no means more *statistically reliable* than it was 40 years ago. The main thing to have changed in the last decades is the standard upon which statistical reliability is based and evaluated. If the fact of the ever-increasing relaxation of these statistical standards of evaluation continues to be ignored, we simply continue to invest in the *fantasy* that psychiatric diagnosis with the DSM is *more reliable than ever before*. Moreover, to this day the plethora of problems addressed by critical researchers in the 1970s (such as the issue of hasty decision-making, and the problems of reification, stigma, and power) remain largely unresolved and, thus, continue to pose a fundamental challenge for contemporary psychiatric diagnosis.

Chapter 3 focuses on how the DSM-5 takes context into account and discusses the kind of entity the DSM considers mental disorders to be. The main argument I make is that in the DSM the context of the individual (i.e., the life history, social circumstances, and cultural background) is thought to play only a minor moderating role in relation to symptom formation and expression. Moreover, as the manual follows a sign-based logic it coheres with the assumption that biological irregularities lie at the basis of mental distress. In this way the DSM cultivates a rather naïve essentialistic view of mental disorders, which is certainly not supported by relevant evidence. In this chapter, starting from phenomenological psychiatry and Lacanian psychoanalysis, I make a plea for a "reflexive" approach to psychopathology. Such an approach does not neglect problem-specific or disorder-specific regularities, but assumes that typical configurations never (unequivocally) apply to single cases, thus demanding a casuistic approach to diagnosis. Starting from the model of symptom formation that was formulated by German Berrios and Ivana Marková I propose a *Triangular Model of Symptom Formation*. Within this model, the symptom is a multidimensional product with certain speech-act specific qualities, biological characteristics, and contextual configuration features covering characteristics that are specific to an individual, family, social context, and (sub-)culture.

Chapter 4 starts with the idea that all diagnostic assessment implies value-laden judgment, and as a result great care must be taken with respect to whose opinions predominate in diagnostic judgment about what is acceptable or not, and what is normal or not. *Psychopathology*, *abnormality*, and *mental disorder* are the core concepts reviewed in this chapter. Starting from Canguilhem it is argued that decision-making about normality and abnormality typically builds on external norms:

conventional opinions of others, like professionals or relatives who believe that some behaviors are not acceptable, or statistical norms that sanction extreme modes of behavior guide this type of judgment. In the diagnosis of psychopathology, the subjective experience of pathos or suffering is central, which I operationalize via the works of Ricoeur on the topic of suffering, and Lacan's distinction between the dimensions of the Real, the Symbolic, and the Imaginary. In this context I make a plea for studying the *quality* of mental suffering in *case formulations* or *case constructions*, which focus on core symptoms and key clinical characteristics in a patient's functioning, and aim to get hold of structural patterns and single incidents that elucidate why an individual functions the way he or she does. Here I indicate that through its focus on mental disorders, and while paying lip service to the idea of taking into account psychopathology, the DSM-5 mainly builds on an assessment of abnormality. To conclude this chapter I contrast two operational ways of dealing with mental suffering in diagnostic contexts. The phenomenological focus of obtaining a genuine understanding of what the patient lives through (*Verstehen*) is juxtaposed with a psychoanalytic approach that states "beware of understanding" (*Gardez-vous de comprendre*), and concentrates on the logic in the patient's functioning.

In Chap. 5 I concentrate on the methodological strengths and pitfalls of clinical case construction, and discuss how the reliability and validity of case formulations can be assured. Chapters 2 and 3 focus on the poor reliability and validity of the DSM. In Chap. 5 I discuss how both methodological dimensions apply to, and can be optimized in, the practice of clinical case construction. Along this way I aim to counter the idea that clinical case construction is less rigorous than psychiatric classification. Starting from clear similarities between the materials used in clinical case formulation, and the data collected by qualitative researchers, I review literature on quality control in qualitative research, and indicate how aspects of it can be used to enhance the quality of clinical case formulation. Three dimensions are discussed: reflexivity, reliability, and validity. I indicate how specific clinical formats that professionals often use (e.g., systematic note taking, case discussions with colleagues, personal therapy, supervision) might function as practices that develop the credibility and confirmability of clinical case formulations.

Shorter versions of the first two chapters of this book were already published in 2014 (*Diagnosis and the DSM—A Critical Review*). Since that time I have further elaborated the lines of reasoning in these chapters, and supplemented them with two further chapters that concentrate on what I consider as an alternative: clinical case formulation. It is my hope that the future of psychiatric and clinical psychological diagnosis is to the personalized and contextualizing approach of clinical case construction.

Other References

Bolton, D. (2013). Overdiagnosis problems in the DSM-IV and the new DSM-5: Can they be resolved by the distress – Impairment criterion? *Canadian Journal of Psychiatry, 58,* 612–617.

Frances, A. (2013). *Saving normal – An insider's revolt against out-of-control psychiatric diagnosis, DSM-5, big pharma, and the medicalization of ordinary life.* New York: William Morrow & Harper Collins Publishers.

Whiteford, H. A., Degenhardt, L., Rehm, J., et al. (2013). Global burden of disease attributable to mental and substance use disorders: Findings from the Global Burden of Disease Study 2010. *The Lancet, 382,* 1575–1586.

World Health Organization. (2013). Mental health action plan 2013–2020. Geneva: World Health Organization. Retrieved June 21, 2016, from http://apps.who.int/iris/bitstream/10665/89966/1/9789241506021_eng.pdf.

2

Dynamics of Decision-Making: The Issue of Reliability in Diagnosis

Diagnosis and the DSM

Publications on diagnosis since the DSM-III often mention the heroic effort made by many in terms of improving its reliability in psychiatry. This is illustrated in the DSM-5 (p. 5), where it states that the "DSM has been the cornerstone of substantial progress in reliability." Indeed, while many proponents of the DSM admit that its validity still poses an unresolved problem, most seem to believe that the manual facilitates a relatively reliable assessment of human suffering. Underlying this line of reasoning is the idea that in the pre-DSM epoch a certain Babylonian confusion of tongues posed problems for psychiatry: different theories existed next to one another, and the concepts used to refer to different disorders were not properly operationally defined, allowing diagnosticians' personal interpretations to strongly guide their diagnostic assessments. With the use of descriptive criteria since DSM-III, all of this changed: finally a sufficiently unambiguous language was found to allow a more rigorous evaluation of observable behaviors. However, the commonly accepted idea of "substantial progress in reliability" is not a proven fact, but an assumption that deserves closer examination.

The issue of reliability is complex and cannot be disconnected from the question of how one thinks of diagnosis as such. In the early days of psychiatric thinking, diagnosis started from prototypes: handbooks described different forms of psychopathology, which were documented with an array of clinical illustrations. Clinicians made use of these prototypical descriptions in assessing and describing the extent to which a given patient's complaints resembled those depicted in the literature, usually ending with categorical assertions on the kind of pathology a patient was suffering from. In this chapter I argue that this prototype-based method of diagnosis lost momentum under the pressure of non-clinical concerns, culminating in a singular focus on classification. The DSM-I (1952) and II (1968) start from prototypes, but reduce prototypical description to a strict minimum, thus illustrating what remains left of diagnosis when classification is its main target. Below I argue that in the 1970s the issue of the reliability of diagnosis became a high priority. During those days, psychiatry was in crisis due to (at least) three important influences: empirical studies began to demonstrate the unreliability of psychiatric decision-making, critical scholars questioned the ethos of psychiatry, and societal changes facilitated a shift toward quantifying mental health policies. The DSM-III (1980) thrived on this crisis and promised a new era of scientific stringency. Prototype-based diagnosis was discredited, while criterion-based diagnosis along the principles of biomedical thinking was hyped. On this point, it is often assumed that since the 1980s psychiatric diagnosis has made great progress. I contend that the statistical reliability of the DSM is seriously overestimated. In 1997 H. Kutchins and S.A. Kirk made such a claim, but the field trials conducted for the DSM-5 in particular illustrate that the "good news parade" on the reliability of the DSM hid its weaknesses for decades. Nevertheless, let us start where it all began and first discuss the shift from prototype-based to criterion-based diagnosis.

From Prototype to Checklist: A Brief History

The checklist-based approach to diagnosis that can be found in the DSM-5 is relatively new to the discipline of psychiatry. Before the DSM-III, psychiatric diagnosis usually started from *prototypes*. At that time, psychiatric handbooks did not contain lists of items, but "clinical pictures": narrative descriptions of different forms of psychopathology. Indeed, the prototypical approach is as old as psychiatry itself and can already be found in the work of the alienist Philippe Pinel. In his book *A Treatise on Insanity,* Pinel (1806) not only reviews key principles of his new discipline, including the moral and medical treatment of insanity, but also provides a study of different "species" of "mental derangement" (Pigeaud 2001). Guided by Immanuel Kant's (1764) suggestion that the diagnostic notions of general medicine might be applied to insanity, and inspired by Thomas Sydenham's (1624–1689) suggestion that diseases should be studied with the method that botanists use in their study of plants, Pinel supposed that *kinds* of insanity could be discerned, hence his belief in the project of collecting a nosology of mental maladies.

In Pinel's view, the insane is subject to all kinds of passions. By observing and listening to patients, writing up their history, and treating them in institutions, he aimed to grasp how passions play a role in different conditions (Pigeaud 2001). Along this way he made distinctions between curable and incurable patients, and between kinds of derangement "depending upon diversities of temperament, habits, intellectual ability, the faculties principally affected, and other causes" (D.D. Davis in: Pinel 1806, p. ii). More specifically, Pinel discerned five forms of mental derangement: melancholia, mania without delirium, mania with delirium, dementia, and idiotism. Melancholia and mania are conditions that were already described since antiquity. Pinel added dementia and idiotism to the list, thus making a classification based on which patients could be categorized. He details these so-called forms of derangement qua the symptoms patients reported as well as clinically observable characteristics. Each specific condition he discerns is marked by distinctive modes of behaving and relating, which he illustrates by means of clinical cases from the Bicêtre Hospital in Paris, as well as historical cases drawn from the literature. Moreover, Pinel aimed to grasp broader patterns underlying specific troubles, such as the typical course and prognosis of a given condition. Obviously Pinel's approach to mental illness focused on describing the original form, or basic type, of the five disorders he discerned; hence the idea that he engendered a *prototypical approach* to diagnosis.

Just like the early botanists made drawings and pictures of the species they discerned, Pinel and his followers described how different kinds of deranged patients characteristically behave, interact, and how they physiognomically looked like.

After Pinel, the prototypical approach long dominated the field of psychiatry. In handbooks outlining different mental illnesses, attention was often paid to the patient's present mental state, patterns at the level of etiology and illness history, and typical prognosis and outcomes. Clinical vignettes of particular patients whose problems fitted in very well with the overall clinical picture were included. Some authors, like Eugen Bleuler (1934), who generally followed an inductive approach to the classification of disorders (Moskowitz and Heim 2011), strongly emphasized the psychological mechanisms connected to specific conditions, like disturbances of association in schizophrenia. Others, like Emil Kraepelin (1921), who followed a more deductive approach, started from biological conjectures (Weber and Engstrom 1997).

The main difference between such a prototype-based approach and the checklist method of the DSM is that diagnosis with prototypes focuses on *sets of characteristics*. Particular behaviors and complaints are not evaluated separately, but examined in terms of *patterns* that make up a person's functioning. Moreover, prototypical diagnosis usually starts from demonstrative cases and clinical vignettes, based on which the clinician evaluates whether a given person's problems match those described in the literature. DSM checklist diagnosis, by contrast, focuses on individual symptoms and signs, leaving aside the question as to how these may relate to one another along an underlying structure. Consequently, the DSM seems to assume that diagnostic criteria are independent of one another and are therefore *additive* in nature. The DSM's additive view on diagnostic criteria is particularly reflected in the DSM-5's severity assessment. Whereas previous versions of the DSM held on to a strict categorical approach, assuming that patients either have a diagnosis or not, the DSM-5 suggests that some disorders manifest in various degrees, depending on the amount of disorder characteristics an individual has. For example, this is illustrated in the DSM-5's (pp. 490–491) category "alcohol use disorder": the more criteria[1] a person meets, the more severe the condition is thought to be. What such an approach leaves out of consideration is the qualitative weight certain characteristics might have: individuals with few symptoms might nevertheless suffer deeply from their condition. Given that mental disorders are defined as disturbances that are associated with "distress or disability" in the DSM-5 (p. 20), the qualitative aspect of subjective suffering in relation to mental symptoms should not be neglected.

The first two editions of the DSM (DSM-I and II) also provided prototypical descriptions of mental disorders, but these descriptions were elaborated very poorly. For example, in the DSM-II (p. 33) schizophrenia is characterized with a paragraph of only 128 words, in which no reference to clinical case material is made. Likewise, subtypes of schizophrenia are described with very brief explanations. For example, the specific description of the hebephrenic type of schizophrenia offers a mere 35 additional words.[2] It mentions clinical characteristics like "disorganized thinking" or "silly and regressive behavior and mannerisms," but doesn't document or operationalize how these typically manifest in clinical practice. References to other authors who might have discussed such characteristics in previous work are also lacking. Compared to the detailed clinical analyses in classic handbooks like that of Bleuler (1934), who devoted 72 pages to his discussion of schizophrenias, the description of specific psychiatric conditions in the early versions of the DSM is extremely concise, and in fact more stereotypical than prototypical in nature.

One reason why the first versions of the DSM were elaborated so poorly is that initially American psychiatrists didn't believe in the relevance of elaborating mere classificatory diagnostic systems (Strand 2011). On the one hand, they had a holistic mental health concept, and assumed that mental illnesses "were precipitated by a combination

---

[1] For alcohol use disorder the DSM-5 (pp. 490–491) lists 11 criteria, including: "Alcohol is often taken in larger amounts or over a longer period than was intended;" "Craving, or a strong desire or urge to use alcohol;" "Recurrent alcohol use in situations in which it is physically hazardous."

[2] "This psychosis is characterized by disorganized thinking, shallow and inappropriate affect, unpredictable giggling, silly and regressive behavior and mannerisms, and frequent hypochondriacal complaints. Delusions and hallucinations, if present, are transient and not well organized" (DSM-II, p. 33).

of psychological and environmental etiological factors that were mediated by the constitution or predisposition of the individual" (Grob 1991, p. 422). On the other hand, they conceived illness in individual terms, which made them focus on the patient rather than on the illness qua abstract category (Grob 1991). For example, Karl Menninger et al. (1958, p. 6) argued that diagnostic labels might well engender an artificial feeling of understanding, but actually don't grasp illness dynamics in patients: "names do not create illness forms; they only comfort the doctors and impress the relatives."

If categorical classification was only of marginal interest to US psychiatrists in the first part of the twentieth century, then why did the American Psychiatric Association decide to publish a handbook like the DSM? The answer to this question cannot be found in the field of clinical psychiatry, but in the work of epidemiologists and statisticians, who aimed to quantify mental distress. In order to make population overviews of different psychiatric conditions they needed straightforward, clearly delineated disorder categories that could be assessed relatively simply.

Serious interest in psychiatric statistics emerged in the mid-nineteenth century, and as large-scale census studies took off in the early twentieth century, the need to develop standardized classification schemes was placed high on the agenda. In 1918 the American Medico-Psychological Association and the US National Committee for Mental Hygiene published the first *Statistical Manual for the Use of Institutions for the Insane*. This manual counts 37 pages and provides a basis for quantitative data collection. It contains sample forms for the administration of patients as well as brief narrative descriptions of 22 mental diseases, spread across 16 pages. Notably, these descriptions are brief, amounting to less than a page. They mainly consist of summaries and descriptions of symptoms and differential diagnostic remarks. Clinical psychiatrists criticized the manual, yet "Despite such criticisms, the *Statistical Manual* became the definitive nosology of the interwar years and went through no fewer than ten editions between 1918 and 1942" (Grob 1991, p. 426). A growing desire to develop a standard nomenclature for psychiatry motivated these revisions. At the side of clinical psychiatry, an impetus to elaborate such classification was found in the work of Emil Kraepelin. While describing and delineating illness entities was a major objective for him, his nosological descriptive approach nevertheless remained strongly narrative in nature.

World War II dramatically changed the overall view of mental disturbance. During these years, severe distress was observed in substantial numbers of soldiers and veterans. Psychoanalytic therapy outside traditional clinics proved to be highly successful in treating these young men, recognizing the link between their distress and the extreme environmental stressors they had been living through (Grob 1991). However, existing classification schemas, like the *Statistical Manual for the Use of Institutions for the Insane* (which was strongly oriented toward residential psychiatry), were of little use in this context: "Only 10 % of the total cases seen [by military psychiatrists] fell into any of the categories ordinarily seen in public mental hospitals" (DSM-I, p. vi). Since neurotic problems and trauma-related psychopathology were not represented in the manual, the US Army and Navy took to developing their own classifications to get hold of the magnitude of mental disorders among soldiers and veterans (Strand 2011). Inspired by both this new classification system and the *Statistical Manual for the Use of Institutions for the Insane*, the American Psychiatric Association made it their business to develop their own statistical manual: the DSM-I was published in 1952. Note that whereas some people seem to believe that the concept "statistical" from the DSM's title refers to statistical evidence that the handbook is based on, this is far from the case. It only indicates that the DSM disorder classes might serve as a basis for categorical classification, and thus provide nominal data for statistical calculations.

The development of the DSM was obviously not really motivated by clinical dilemmas, but by *administrative concerns*: bureaucrats and social scientists alike wanted to obtain statistics about mental health problems. The net effect of adopting such classificatory systems was that the concept "diagnosis" was narrowed down quite dramatically. Etymologically the concept "diagnosis" (from the Greek "diagignoskein") refers to "discern" as well as to "know thoroughly" (Harper 2011). In the context of the DSM, diagnosis is not so much concerned with *developing thorough knowledge* about an individual's mental health conditions, like traditional clinical psychiatrists were. From the outset, it simply focused on *distinguishing* between different disorders. Indeed, from its inception the DSM largely equated diagnosis with classification, leaving aside the elaborate narrative description of a patient's global functioning. This is a reduction that remains neglected. This reduction is productive if one wants to quantify human problems, as it opens the possibility of statistical computation. However, this leaves us with the very serious question as to whether such a leaning toward categorization facilitates an accurate characterization of an individual's mental suffering.

Indeed, as I further explain in Chap. 3, it could be argued that from its inception the DSM approached psychopathology in a naturalistic way, thus neglecting the subjective experience of psychopathology and above all its contextual embedment. Eventually, the DSM-I contained 106 disorders, a notable increase from the 22 disorders outlined in the 1918 *Statistical Manual for the Use of Institutions for the Insane*. As is true for all subsequent editions of the DSM, arguments and evidence that substantiated this fivefold increase in the number of disorders were not published in the DSM or in related sources.[3] As a result, it remains unclear as to what motives and interests guided these revisions. Overall, the DSM-I distinguishes between brain disorders, mental deficiency, psychotic disorders, psychophysiologic disorders, psychoneurotic disorders, personality disorders, and adjustment reactions. These are defined by short descriptors across a total of 42 pages. Next to that, the handbook contains sections with guidelines and classification forms for statistical analysis, also spanning 42 pages.

As the DSM-I was adopted in the 1950s, diagnostic classification remained a marginal concern to the then dominant group of psychodynamic psychiatrists in the USA (Strand 2011). Often, generic psychiatric labels, like schizophrenia or melancholia, were seen to be too imprecise as characterizations for grasping the problems a patient suffers from. For example, Karl Menninger (1959) argued that mere classification is insufficient. In his view a psychiatric diagnosis "is always a complex set of statements – descriptive, analytic and evaluative. They have

---

[3] It could be argued that as such, an increase in the number of mental disorders is not necessarily negative: it could indicate that the profession developed a more refined understanding of mental disorders, and thus made an evolution in the direction of more precise diagnosis. However, as we discuss in Chap. 3, the validity of most DSM categories was, and is, problematic: the numerical increase of diagnostic categories does not rest on solid grounds.

to describe a patient's method of interacting with his environment, past and present [...] and the psychiatric diagnosis is always both polydimensional and multidisciplinary" (Menninger 1959, pp. 233–234). Such focus on the case-specific study of the meaning and function of symptoms changed only slightly when the American Psychiatric Association was asked to attune the manual to the standards outlined by the *International Classification of Diseases* (ICD). In 1948 the international community, under the auspices of the United Nations, created the World Health Organization (WHO). One of the objectives of the WHO was to standardize medical classification. Its tool for realizing this objective was the ICD, which provides a taxonomic list of all recognized forms of medical illness. At first, the ICD listed only somatic diseases, but in 1949 a section on mental disorders was added. Given the membership of the USA to the WHO, the American Psychiatric Association was asked to attune its diagnostic system to the ICD format. This gave rise to the DSM-II (1968), an elaboration of the DSM-I, which comprises 182 disorders. Indeed, between 1952 and 1968 the number of diagnoses again increased substantially, but overall, the DSM-II didn't differ much from the elementary prototypical approach of the DSM-I.

Finally, in 1980, with the publication of the DSM-III, the American Psychiatric Association dropped its elementary prototype-based approach for a checklist-based system, a system that can still be found in the DSM-5. The main reasons for this switch is likely rooted in the harsh discussions on the fundaments and the practice of psychiatry during the 1960s and 1970s (Decker 2013). During these years, as mentioned earlier, psychiatry was in crisis. In response to this discontent, a restoration movement took shape that was somewhat opposed to psychodynamic theory and practice. A group of so-called neo-Kraepelinian psychiatrists at Washington University in St. Louis responded to the malaise in the discipline by defining psychiatry more strongly as a strictly medical discipline (Decker 2007, 2013). This group heavily influenced the revisions that gave rise to the DSM-III and provided psychiatry with a redefinition of its object. During the decades in which psychoanalysis was the dominant framework, much attention was paid to unconscious conflict, object relations, and drive-related dynamics in different types of psychopathology. The neo-Kraepelinians shied away from the psychoanalytic discourse, firmly steering toward the use of biomedical concepts and methods with respect to the study and treatment of mental illness. Indeed, as M. Strand (2011) indicates, the principal motive in this shift toward the checklist-based system of the DSM-III can be found in an effort toward "ontological transmutation": psychiatrists aimed to redefine the controversial object of psychiatry by firmly connecting it to medical discourse. More than ever before, diagnostic classification preceding psychiatric and psychological treatment became a central concern. Below I review how and why this transition took shape in greater detail, focusing on studies that demonstrated the unreliability of prototype-based psychiatric diagnosis.

Commotion in Psychiatry, Part I: Diagnosis Under Fire in the 1970s

The reason why psychiatry was contested in the late 1960s and 1970s is illustrated in a series of critical empirical studies that documented the poor reliability and validity of psychiatric diagnosis. I illustrate this below through three iconic studies.

The first study was conducted by Maurice Temerlin (1968, 1970). In 1968 Temerlin published a paper on a naturalistic experimental study in which he asked 25 psychiatrists, 25 clinical psychologists, and 45 clinical psychology students to diagnose an individual. Participants listened to an audiotaped interview with an actor who followed a script, that of a normal, healthy man. However, prior to listening to the recording an eminent colleague remarked that the individual they were about to hear was "a very interesting man because he looked neurotic but actually was quite psychotic" (Temerlin 1968, p. 1949). After listening to the recording, participants were asked to indicate their diagnosis on a data-sheet containing multiple diagnostic categories: "10 psychoses, 10 neuroses and 10 miscellaneous personality types, one of which was 'normal or healthy personality'" (Temerlin 1968, p. 350). Moreover, they were asked to substantiate their diagnosis by noting down the behavioral characteristics that guided them in their decision.

The result was quite shocking: 15 psychiatrists gave a diagnosis of psychosis, while 10 concluded that they were dealing with a case of neurosis. The clinical psychologists were slightly more precise in their decision: 7 diagnosed psychosis, 15 neurosis, and 3 indicated that he was normal. The graduate students, in their turn, were the most accurate: 5 indicated that the interviewee was psychotic, 35 pointed to neurosis, and 5 believed he was in good mental health.

In the next step, the study was replicated in three control conditions. First, the interview was presented with reverse suggestion, that is, with an eminent colleague saying that the man on the tape is normal. All 20 mental health professionals participating in this condition agreed that he was normal. In the second control condition, the interview was presented without suggestion to a group of 21 mental health professionals. This time no one indicated that the interviewee was psychotic: 9 believed he was neurotic and 12 that he was normal. In the third control condition, the tape was presented to 12 laypersons. Again, no suggestion was made, and all of them agreed that the interviewee was in good mental health. When Temerlin finally studied the participants' written notes he observed that only the participants who arrived at making a correct diagnosis made good résumés. Indeed, only those who characterized the interviewee as normal provided accurate paraphrasing of what the actor had actually said. Others either made very poor summaries or mentioned personal inferences rather than observations.

Overall, Temerlin concluded that diagnostic appraisals made by psy-professionals were highly influenced by prejudice and suggestion. This influence is situated at two levels. First, the huge impact of the eminent colleague's informal comment shows that trained professionals' decision-making was not guided by strong internal standards: they were exceedingly suggestible and proved to be biased by a variety of contextual influences. Second, the difference between the professionals and the laypersons in the non-suggestion condition illustrates that specialized knowledge did not aid them in drawing valid conclusions, but instead engendered a certain prejudice. After all, while the script was highly balanced and did not contain references to symptoms, mental suffering, or underlying psychopathological processes, almost half of the professionals in the non-suggestion condition believed that the interviewee had some kind of neurosis. Finally, the participants' observation notes were far from accurate. They contained elements of prejudice and misrepresentation that subsequently distorted their evaluation. Indeed, the major impact of prejudice and suggestion not only implies that the reliability of psychiatric decision-making is low, but more importantly indicates that the validity of psychiatric diagnosis was fundamentally questionable.

The Temerlin study came as a bombshell: highly qualified professionals who were enveloped by an aura of seriousness suddenly proved to be simply uncritical and biased in their lines of reasoning: emperors without clothes. Without explicitly referring to the Temerlin study, in 1973 clinical psychologist Paul Meehl further substantiated this problem. In his influential essay "Why I Do Not Attend Case Conferences," Meehl listed several weaknesses in how the clinical decision-making process, at that time, often took shape in psychiatric settings. His list is impressive and further demonstrates why the then common practices of informal data gathering and diagnostic decision-making were not only inadequate, but sometimes blatantly erroneous. Problems he reviews include the following:

- The use of low standards in evaluating the quality of clinical evidence, as a result of which mere anecdotes have an equal status as carefully collected data, and irrelevant details tend to prevail over crucial features;
- A lack of critical thinking and true debate among practitioners, especially when their own cases are discussed;
- Sloppy adherence to rules of scientific inference, logical decision-making, and probabilistic thinking;
- The custom usage of fallacies that compromise the decision-making process, including the Barnum effect (saying trivial things about a case that are true for almost everyone), the sick-sick fallacy (people very unlike me are seen as sick), the me-too fallacy (people that resemble me are seen as healthy), and the ad hoc fallacy (using after-the-fact causal explanations);

- The inadequate use or plain neglect of essential psychiatric textbook knowledge, for example, in drawing differential diagnostic conclusions;
- The hasty use of complex theoretical speculations in making sense of elementary case materials.

Taken together these problems, which Meehl (1973) described as so common that attending clinical case meetings was no longer worth the effort, provided a shocking picture of clinical psychiatric practice: rather than being informed by scientific methods and insights, diagnostic decision-making seemed governed by all kinds of flaws.

The second iconic study, which further demonstrated a number of problems mentioned by Meehl, was published by David Rosenhan in the highly prestigious journal *Science* (1973, 1975). In order to test how professionals appraise minimal psychiatric symptoms, Rosenhan recruited eight individuals without psychiatric problems, "sane people" (1973, p. 179), and sent them as pseudo-patients to 12 hospitals in total. The pseudo-patients contacted the hospitals with the complaint that they were hearing voices that were communicating ambiguous messages, like "empty," "hollow," and "thud." Aside from providing information about these voices, the pseudo-patients did not give any other information related to (psycho)pathology and answered all further questions truthfully: "Beyond alleging the symptoms and falsifying name, vocation, and employment, no further alterations of person, history, or circumstances were made" (Rosenhan 1973, p. 180). All participants were admitted to the hospital, at which moment they ceased feigning any further characteristics of abnormality. Rosenhan was interested in how the pseudo-patients would be diagnosed, and observed that after an average of 19 days of hospitalization the participants were discharged with the following diagnoses: 11 with a diagnosis of schizophrenia and 1 with a diagnosis of manic-depressive psychosis, all of them with the added specification of "in remission." Rosenhan concluded that the diagnoses were not based on the relative normality of the pseudo-patients or their behavior in the ward. Rather, the fact of staying in a hospital provided a context in which minor symptoms were magnified and normal behaviors were pathologized, illustrating the sick-sick fallacy coined by Meehl

(1973). Rosenhan anecdotally substantiated this conclusion by referring to a case summary prepared by one hospital as their pseudo-patient was discharged. In line with Meehl's (1973) observation that clinicians tend to rapidly make use of complex theoretical speculations, often getting trapped in the ad hoc fallacy, the case report "explained" the hallucinatory symptom by referring to affective instability and ambivalence in the pseudo-patient's family constellation; this, it was concluded, had provoked a schizophrenic reaction. With this experiment, Rosenhan set the problem of false-positive diagnosis (i.e., giving a diagnosis when it is unwarranted) on the agenda of scholars in psychiatry.

When Rosenhan first presented his results, the general response in the psychiatric establishment was disbelief. One hospital reacted that such frank errors would never occur in their institution, and to test this brave assertion, Rosenhan (1973, 1975) introduced a second phase to his experiment. He told the hospital that in the next three months one or more pseudo-patients would again attempt to get admitted to the hospital. Each staff member was asked to rate incoming patients according to the likelihood that they were pseudo-patients. Judgments were obtained on 193 admitted patients. The results seemed promising: 42 admitted patients were qualified, with unflinching confidence, as pseudo-patients by at least one staff member; 23 were alleged to be pseudo-patients according to their psychiatrist; and 19 were alleged to be pseudo-patients according to the psychiatrist and at least one other member of staff. Hospital staff were now meticulous in their detection of what could be false-positive diagnoses. The only problem in all of this is that Rosenhan had not actually sent anyone to the hospital. Indeed, the second phase of the experiment casted even more doubt on the validity of psychiatric diagnosis, and put the credibility of psychiatric practice into question.

Rosenhan's second experiment opened up at least two possible interpretations. On the one hand, the results demonstrated the danger of false-negative diagnosis (giving no diagnosis when it seems justified). On the other hand, Rosenhan's findings could be interpreted as a fundamental attack on psychiatry, as such: if staff had serious doubts about the authenticity of the complaints in 10–20 % of their patients, why did they decide to treat them in a residential setting? What is more, questions on the quality of psychiatric treatment also came to the fore in notes made by the participants in the first phase of the experiment. Based on their daily observations in the ward, staff were characterized as disinterested in the patients' problems. Occasionally staff members displayed basic misconduct in relation to patients and overall developed relationships whereby the patients felt powerless and were treated impersonally.

Rosenhan's study aroused debate about the discipline of psychiatry, as well as criticism by colleagues. Robert Spitzer, the president of the DSM-III task force, expressed one such criticism, using Rosenhan's study to actually promote diagnosis that utilized standardized checklists (Spitzer 1975, pp. 450–452). In his view, the Rosenhan experiments were mere pseudo-science in *Science*. Contrary to the common interpretation of the results, Spitzer (1975) suggested that the psychiatrists were actually correct in their consideration of psychosis. After all, the hallucinations might have indicated an acute schizophrenic episode, concerning which the DSM-II (p. 34) specifies that "in many cases the patient recovers within weeks." The psychiatrists were correct when they described the condition as "in remission": "The meaning of 'in remission' is clear: it means without signs of illness. Thus, all of the psychiatrists apparently recognized that all of the pseudo-patients were, to use Rosenhan's term, 'sane'" (Spitzer 1975, p. 444). As he examined actual patient files from hospitals, Spitzer observed that the diagnosis "in remission" was used very rarely. The fact that it was used in Rosenhan's study thus demonstrates that psychiatrists were actually very accurate in their evaluation. Meanwhile the damage had been done to the image of psychiatric diagnosis.

Actually, Spitzer himself was a key figure in pointing to severe methodological problems with psychiatric diagnosis. Together with a collaborating statistician, Joseph Fleiss, he published a third iconic study, in which he argued that problems with inter-rater reliability in habitual prototypical diagnosis were insurmountable (Spitzer and Fleiss 1974). With the aim of making a comprehensive overview of diagnostic reliability they aggregated data from six major studies that examined how well diagnosticians usually reach agreement in their evaluation of the same patient. All studies included were published between the late 1950s and 1970s. The accumulated data included 1726 patients, all diagnosed by two psychiatrists. The diagnostic system used in the six studies differed slightly, but allowed aggregation in terms of the DSM-II disorder categories. Spitzer and Fleiss checked inter-rater agreement by calculating a *kappa statistic* for each DSM-II disorder category. This statistic *estimates* agreement between judges, but incorporates a correction for agreement based on mere chance. As Diana E. Clarke et al. (2013, p. 47) indicate, kappa coefficients reflect "the difference between the probabilities of getting a second positive diagnosis between those with a first positive and those with a first negative diagnosis."

The next paragraphs in this section provide a methodological discussion of the study by Spitzer and Fleiss. Some parts might be hard to follow for those who are not particularly interested in numbers. However, a detailed discussion of reliability studies dating from the 1970s is important for an accurate evaluation of the idea that with the publication of DSM-III the reliability of psychiatric diagnoses strongly improved.

In a nutshell, what Spitzer and Fleiss attempted to argue was that in the 1960s and 1970s psychiatric diagnosis was not reliable. However, as I outline below, their method of reaching this conclusion started from rather high evaluation thresholds for the kappa statistic, making poor reliability results more likely. Indeed, it was on the basis of these high standards for the kappa statistic that poor reliability was established. This appears to have given the authors reasonable grounds to denounce the classic prototype-based method of diagnosis, which we saw characterized the method of diagnosis of the previous decades, and ultimately argue for a switch to the checklist format, that is, that which characterizes the DSM-III and subsequent editions of the manual. As we will see, reliability studies on the DSM-III (and its successors) indicate that diagnostic reliability improved substantially over the years. However, as I hope to demonstrate, this conclusion is spurious: whereas the *magnitude* of the kappa coefficients largely remained the same over the years, what seems to have changed was the *threshold* for which they were being interpreted.

While strict norms for interpreting the kappa coefficient do not exist, several authors have presented standards for interpreting them. In an early paper on the kappa statistic Fleiss and Cohen (1973) devoted a section to the interpretation of the kappa coefficient. At that moment, no fixed standards for using the statistic seemed to have been established, yet the authors suggested that the kappa coefficient could be interpreted as an intra-class correlation coefficient. In another paper, Spitzer and colleagues argued that numerical scales of psychopathology "typically have reliabilities in the interval 0.70 to 0.90," which motivated Spitzer and Fleiss (1974) to use this interval to evaluate the values of the kappa statistics collected: reliability is high if the coefficient is more than 0.90, satisfactory if it falls in the 0.70– 0.90 range, and unacceptable if the obtained coefficient is lower than 0.70.

However, over the years, commonly accepted standards for interpreting the kappa coefficient were reformulated, whereby norms for evaluating it relaxed considerably. For example, J.R. Landis and G.G. Koch (1977) proposed to adhere to one frequently used standard: They cautiously indicate that a kappa value of more than 0.75 indicates excellent reliability, while a value between 0.40 and 0.75 points to fair to good reliability, and a value below 0.40 is indicative of poor reliability. In 1981 Spitzer's collaborator Joseph Fleiss endorsed these more flexible norms. He proposed to use them to interpret kappa coefficients (Fleiss et al. 1981, p. 609), and thus to leave aside the previously formulated standard that used a 0.70 to 0.90 interval. Later on, further refinement in the interpretation of the kappa coefficient was argued for. Indeed, the standards that were used to interpret the DSM-5 field trial data (Clarke et al. 2013), which we discuss later, delineate kappa values of 0.80 and above as excellent, indicating almost perfect agreement; values from 0.60 to 0.79 as very good, indicating substantial agreement; kappa values from 0.40 to 0.59 as good, indicating moderate agreement; values from 0.20 to 0.39 as questionable, indicating fair agreement; and values below 0.20 as unacceptable, indicating slight agreement (see also Kraemer et al. 2002; Viera and Garrett 2005).[4] An overview of these sets of kappa evaluation standards[5] can be found in Table 2.1. Balanced evaluations of results from

---

[4] Other contemporary statisticians hold on to more strict norms for the kappa statistic. Baer and Blais (2010) suggest that kappa values > 0.70 are excellent; values between 0.60 and 0.70 are good; values between 0.41 and 0.59 are questionable; and values ≤ 0.40 are poor. Considered from these standards, the norms used in the DSM-5 field trial are unacceptably generous (Vanheule et al. 2014).

[5] Kappa values are estimated based on a formula in which different parameters are taken into account. Imagine a situation in which 2 judges rate 100 patients with 2 classification possibilities

Table 2.1 Overview of three sets of norms for evaluating the kappa statistic

Authors	Cut-off points
Spitzer and Fleiss (1974)	≥ 0.90: excellent 0.70– 0.90: satisfactory ≤ 0.70: unacceptable
Landis and Koch (1977)	≥ 0.75: excellent 0.40– 0.75: fair too good ≤ 0.40: poor
Clarke et al. (2013)	≥ 0.80: excellent 0.60– 0.79: very good 0.40– 0.59: good 0.20– 0.39: questionable ≤ 0.20: unacceptable

inter-rater reliability studies that were conducted throughout the years should take into account these changing norms. Indeed, this important evolution in statistical standards of evaluation seems to have been largely ignored. In other words, over time, the standards upon which statistical evaluations were made relaxed substantially. If these changes are not taken into account, the results of different studies simply cannot be compared.

In interpreting their aggregated data from reliability studies published between the late 1950s and early 1970s, Spitzer and Fleiss (1974) used the strict standard they themselves formulated (see Table 2.2). This brought them to the conclusion that the reliability of pre-DSM-III diagnosis was disappointing. Indeed, as one applies their norms none of the diagnostic categories has high reliability: no coefficients are higher than 0.90. Only three diagnostic categories fall into the 0.70 to 0.90 interval for acceptable reliability (i.e., "mental deficiency, organic brain syndrome (but not its subtypes), and alcoholism" (Spitzer and Fleiss 1974, p. 344)). For 15 out of the 18 studied diagnostic categories, by contrast, kappa values were below 0.70, meaning that for these

---

(e.g., psychotic versus not psychotic). In this case, starting from Cohen's formula, a kappa value of 0 indicates that both judges agree in 50 % of the cases, which is as much as one would expect based on coincidence. A kappa value of 0.25 in its turn means that they agree on about 62 % of the cases; 0.50 means agreement on 75 % of the cases; 0.75 means agreement on about 87 % of the cases. If parameters change, the corresponding percentages also slightly change. For example, in a situation where two judges rate 100 patients starting from five classification possibilities a kappa value of 0 indicates that both judges agree in 20 %of the cases; 0.25 means agreement on 40 % of the cases; 0.50 means agreement on 60 % of the cases; 0.75 means agreement on 80 % of the cases.

Table 2.2 Kappa coefficients for DSM-II categories, adapted from Spitzer and Fleiss (1974, p. 344), and three sets of interpretations of the Kappa coefficient using different norms

Disorder category	Kappa	Interpretation Spitzer and Fleiss (1974) norms	Interpretation Landis and Koch (1977) norms	Interpretation Clarke et al. (2013) norms
Mental deficiency	0.72	Satisfactory	Fair to good	Very good
Organic brain syndrome	0.77	Satisfactory	Excellent	Very good
Acute brain syndrome	0.44	Unacceptable	Fair to good	Good
Chronic brain syndrome	0.64	Unacceptable	Fair to good	Very good
Alcoholism	0.71	Satisfactory	Fair to good	Very good
Psychosis	0.55	Unacceptable	Fair to good	Good
Schizophrenia	0.57	Unacceptable	Fair to good	Good
Affective disorder	0.41	Unacceptable	Fair to good	Good
Neurotic depression	0.26	Unacceptable	Poor	Questionable
Psychotic depression	0.24	Unacceptable	Poor	Questionable
Manic-depressive	0.33	Unacceptable	Poor	Questionable
Involutional depression	0.30	Unacceptable	Poor	Questionable
Personality disorder or neurosis	0.44	Unacceptable	Fair to good	Good
Personality disorder	0.32	Unacceptable	Poor	Questionable
Sociopathic	0.53	Unacceptable	Fair to good	Good
Neurosis	0.40	Unacceptable	Fair to good	Good
Anxiety reaction	0.45	Unacceptable	Fair to good	Good
Psychophysiological reaction	0.38	Unacceptable	Poor	Questionable

conditions reliabilities were unacceptable. This brought the authors to the following conclusion: "The reliability of psychiatric diagnosis as it has been practiced since at least the late 1950s is not good" (Spitzer and Fleiss 1974, p. 345). What is remarkable about Spitzer and Fleiss's (1974) paper is that they act as if the norms they applied were commonly accepted, while in reality this was not the case. This might indicate that they were either very naive in their use of the kappa coefficient, or they were determined to finish with psychiatric diagnosis, as commonly practiced between the late 1950s and the early 1970s. Reading their 1974 paper today, it seems they, above all, aimed at paving the way for checklist-based diagnosis. After all, following their general conclusion that the quality of psychiatric diagnosis was poor, Spitzer and Fleiss (1974) suggested that an overall change in the practice of diagnosis was needed. Referring to an older study by Aaron Beck et al. (1962), which demonstrated that diagnostic unreliability was mainly due to ambiguities in commonly used nomenclature, they suggested that the descriptions of disorders in the DSM-II were far too imprecise, and that a different method of diagnosis was necessary. The alternative method they proposed was indeed the checklist approach Spitzer embedded in the DSM-III.

However, if one interprets the kappa coefficients collected by Spitzer and Fleiss (1974) using the norms proposed by Landis and Koch (1977), a different conclusion comes to the fore (see Table 2.2). Based on their standards, reliability is excellent for 1 diagnostic category: organic brain disorder; fair to good for 11 diagnostic categories; and poor for 6 categories, including the subtypes of depression, personality disorder, and psychophysiological reaction. Indeed, bearing in mind Landis and Koch's (1977) norms, strong assertions like those made by Spitzer and Fleiss (1974) cannot be confirmed, since two-thirds of the diagnostic categories show fair to excellent reliabilities. For example, applying these norms one can conclude that the diagnostic reliability of the classic diagnostic categories, neurosis and psychosis, is fine. In view of the harsh discussions around the diagnostic category of neurosis during the development of the DSM-III, this might sound ironic. Indeed, as Hannah Decker (2013) documented extremely well, the category of neurosis was a divisive element in the late 1970s when the DSM-III was composed: psychoanalysts were convinced that neurosis was a crucial concept in diagnostic work, while biomedically inspired psychiatrists believed it was a useless category because of its link with psychoanalytic theory. The psychoanalysts lost the debate. Among other reasons, psychoanalysts' staunch attitude and poor knowledge of statistics and research methods have been their undoing: they couldn't detect the holes in Spitzer's methodology, and failed to substantiate the credibility of the neurosis concept. It was thus deleted as a diagnostic category. In the DSM-III the term "neurosis" was relegated to a few disorder category subtitles, and this as a descriptive label only. Eventually the concept disappeared from the later editions of the handbook.

As one interprets the kappa coefficients from the Spitzer and Fleiss (1974) study with the kappa norms used in the DSM-5 field trial (Clarke et al. 2013), the interpretation is even more positive: very good reliability for four categories; good reliability for eight categories, including neurosis, psychosis and affective disorder; and questionable reliability for the six categories that Landis and Koch's (1977) standard had also evaluated as poor. Indeed, the use of contemporary norms provides a completely different picture of the reliability of pre-DSM-III diagnosis. Starting from Spitzer and Fleiss's (1974) benchmarks, the reliability was unacceptable for 15 of the 18 disorder categories. In terms of contemporary standards, by contrast, none of the diagnostic categories has an unacceptably low reliability: for 12 disorders reliability is good to very good, and for six categories inter-rater reliability is questionable.

However, history teaches us that until now the interpretation by Spitzer and Fleiss (1974) set the tone. Their interpretation substantiated the idea that in the 1970s psychiatric diagnosis was in deep crisis, and that drastic reforms were necessary. In the discussion of their paper Spitzer and Fleiss (1974) not only proposed a switch to checklist-based thinking, but also implied that diagnostic categories with psychoanalytic origins, like neurosis, caused diagnostic unreliability, which is why Spitzer campaigned against these categories and eventually strived to remove them from the DSM-III (Decker 2013). Spitzer himself was initially trained in psychoanalysis, but disliked the method, believing that by switching to a biomedical model psychiatry could make great advances.

In later publications, neither Spitzer nor any other officials working on subsequent editions of the DSM pointed to the evolution in the use of the kappa statistic, meaning that the early claims of Spitzer and Fleiss (1974) were never properly put into perspective. Based on their results Spitzer and Fleiss simply denounced diagnosis based on prototypes, and, as we will argue later on in this chapter, made a plea for a biomedical approach to psychopathology. Interestingly, recent research demonstrates that the idea that the prototype-based method diagnosis is unreliable is untenable. For example, Drew Westen and associates launched and tested a prototype-matching approach to diagnosis: "diagnosticians compare a patient's overall clinical presentation to a set of diagnostic prototypes – for clinical use, paragraph-length descriptions of empirically identified disorders – and rate the 'goodness of fit' or extent of match of the patient's clinical presentation to the prototype" (2012, p. 17). Applied to the diagnosis of mood and anxiety disorders, such prototype-based diagnoses cohered with consistent patterns among criterion variables, and were actually better in predicting self-reported symptoms than DSM-based categorical diagnosis (DeFife et al. 2013). Applied to personality disorders this method yielded highly reliable judgments: in an inter-rater reliability study including 65 patients a median correlation of 0.72 was observed (Westen et al. 2010). In a study focusing on 62 adolescent psychiatric patients a mean correlation of 0.70 was observed (Haggerty et al. 2016). However, in the 1970s researchers in psychiatry concluded that prototype-based diagnosis was unreliable and that a switch to a checklist-based approach was needed.

Commotion in Psychiatry, Part II: Critical Researchers Dethrone the Psychiatric Ethos

In the 1960s and 1970s psychiatry was not only challenged by studies on the unreliability of psychiatric diagnosis. The discipline was also in crisis because researchers in the social sciences and the humanities looked at psychiatry from new and increasingly critical perspectives. Several scholars are noteworthy, such as sociologist Thomas Scheff (1966), whose work on labeling shed a new light on diagnosis, and psychiatrist Ronald D. Laing (1960), who assumed that symptoms of mental illness express concerns one cannot communicate. Nevertheless, here we focus two other scholars from fairly different research traditions: Thomas Szasz and Michel Foucault.

A first key figure who, in the 1960s and 1970s, strongly criticized the commonly accepted models of diagnosis was psychiatrist Thomas Szasz. The basic idea he put forth in his 1961 monograph *The Myth of Mental Illness* is that until then psychiatric thinking was too focused on "thinking in terms of substantives." This means that in his view, psychiatric problems were too strongly thought of as deeply ingrained conditions, while "process-thinking," which focuses on dynamical processes, was neglected (Szasz 1961, p. 2). Process-thinking is interactional in nature, and explores how problems are constructed within contexts. Szasz suggests that as long as it is not proven that psychiatric symptoms are actually caused by underlying biological deficits, it makes no sense to interpret them as signs of medical illness. Focusing on the example of hysterical complaints, he suggests that, first and foremost, psychiatric symptoms have a communicative function. Hysterical complaints are proto-linguistic communications that follow the language of organic disease, but, as symptoms, they have to be deciphered. In his view, psychiatric symptoms should be studied in terms of people's sign-using behavior. Starting from game theory, Szasz aimed to isolate the underlying rules that govern patterns associated with symptomatic behaviors. In order to substantiate his point, Szasz (1961) documents how different contexts, for example, nineteenth versus twentieth century, or the USA versus the former Soviet Union, entail different forms of symptomatic expression. If psychiatric symptoms were stable biologically rooted entities, this kind of contextual variation should have no substantial impact, while this impact is indeed present. He therefore concludes that "the search for the physical causation of many so-called psychological phenomena may be motivated more by the prestige-need of the investigators than by a quest of scientific clarity" (Szasz 1961, p. 81). So what is at the root of psychiatric symptoms? Szasz (1961, p. 75) believes they comprise "problems of human living – or of existence" that are communicated by proto-linguistic signs. For example, a person might be disappointed in life, and experience certain events as a "slap in the face" in the figurative sense, but instead of communicating disappointment he might start experiencing facial pain, which is then communicated to others. Facial pain expresses the disappointment, but doesn't communicate it verbally, hence the idea that it is a primitive proto-linguistic communication: "It makes communication concerning a significant subject possible, while at the same time it helps the speaker to disown the disturbing implications of his message" (Szasz 1961, p. 124). This communicative process is largely unconscious and disturbs human interaction if not properly understood.

Indeed, on the one hand, Szasz's book, which focuses on hysterical complaints, might be interpreted as a plea for an interaction-based relational model of psychopathology. In the DSM-II hysterical complaints are classified as psychophysiological reactions. This is one of the diagnostic categories with low inter-rater reliability in the study by Spitzer and Fleiss (1974). Szasz's book, therefore, might be seen as an attempt to get hold of these Janus-head symptoms, but by following a relational-communicative approach instead of a biological approach. On the other hand, however, the provocative tone of this book might also be taken up as an anti-psychiatric attack on the biomedical model. He calls psychiatrists "pseudo physicians" who are "striving for prestige by aping the 'natural scientists'"[6] (Szasz 1961, p. 82). In terms of Szasz's (1961) own theory, such bold assertions are "rule-breaking communications," which have a predictable effect: the establishment was offended and Szasz's point was completely lost in the midst of all the commotion. Indeed, for many, his message was likely taken as pure heresy. Nevertheless, it is arguable that more than half a century later, many of the points Szasz put forward still hold true. If one accepts, as Szasz (1961) assumed, "that illness involves a deviation from the normal anatomical or physiological structure and functioning of the human body," one could conclude, as Hanna Pickard (2009, p. 84) suggests, that this does not hold for most mental disorders.

A second key figure in critical discussions on psychiatry was French philosopher and historian Michel Foucault. In his 1965 book *Madness and Civilization: A History of Insanity in the Age of Reason*[7] Foucault analyzes how society dealt with insanity throughout history, focusing on the Renaissance, the seventeenth and eighteenth centuries, and modern times. The point he makes is that whereas in the Middle Ages the so-called *madman* was a figure inside society, subsequent epochs defined him as an outsider. From then on, the *insane* person was an outcast that must be confined; a sick individual that should be studied and treated as

---

[6] In his later work, Szasz again chose the path of provocation. Combined with his controversial libertarian views he ended up alienating many people in the fields of psychiatry and psychoanalysis.
[7] The English edition published in 1964 is an abbreviated version of Foucault's original work from 1961.

a medical object. Key to this historical evolution was the creation of asylums at the end of the eighteenth century, for instance, by Pinel, where the madman was treated by a new category of medical doctors, namely, alienists, who above all functioned as authority figures. At first this subjection was explicit in the practice of moral treatment, which subjected the unreasonable insane to the *discipline* of the reasonable medical doctor. In the late eighteenth century, as positivism imposed itself upon medicine and psychiatry, this disciplinary power relation became less visible. It was still present but veiled under a naturalizing discourse that was henceforth used to explain madness (Kirsher 2009).

As a consequence, in Foucault's (1965, p. 276) view madness is not so much a natural kind, that is, an entity governed by natural laws, but what he calls "a reification of a magical nature." In his view, psychiatry did not arise because medical doctors had suddenly discovered an underlying biomedical reality that could be linked to the behaviors of the so-called insane. On the contrary, psychiatry came into existence as it brought its own object into being: disciplinary practices first delineated a group of outcasts that were amenable for adaptation to society, and later defined them as proper objects for scientific study: "What we call psychiatric practice is a certain moral tactic contemporary with the end of the eighteenth century, preserved in the rites of asylum life, and overlaid by the myths of positivism" (Foucault 1965, p. 267). By qualifying madness as a *reification* Foucault stresses that the early alienists, just like modern psychiatrists, *turned their concept into an object*. As a consequence "madness" was no longer treated as an abstraction that can be used to make sense of the world, but as a biological or psychological reality that simply awaits clinical detection and scientific discovery. Such reification is a direct effect of adopting psychiatric discourse. Through the use of specific language, the concept under discussion is materialized, or as Friedrich Nietzsche (1887, p. 122) put it: "it is enough to create new names and estimations and probabilities in order to create in the long run new 'things.'"

Meanwhile this notion of reification slowly became recognized as a problem in psychiatry. What is more, DSM-based diagnosis in particular was at last accused of promulgating such reification (Nieweg 2005), thus giving rise to what Steven Hyman (2010, p. 157), a former president of the US National Institute of Mental Health, calls "an unintended epistemic prison." Indeed, while the diagnostic categories of the DSM are nothing but conventional groupings of symptoms or "heuristics that have proven extremely useful in clinical practice and research" (Hyman 2010, p. 156), people still tend to think of them as real entities. For example, reification is evident when people think of "ADHD" or "schizophrenia" as underlying diseases that give rise to characteristic symptoms, while in fact these labels are nothing but descriptive umbrella terms used to designate a collection of symptoms that make up particular syndromes. Reification produces the added problem of the so-called disorders being understood as quasi-material conditions that *cause* symptoms, while in fact they only indicate that a (certain) minimal number of category-specific symptoms have been observed in an individual. In other words, DSM diagnoses do not *explain* anything beyond this idle descriptive classification, yet people tend to invest belief in them as real entities, which is clearly absurd. While they didn't use the concept, the effect of reification that is associated with labeling psychiatric disorders also seems the point Karl Menninger et al. (1958, p. 6) had in mind when arguing that names for illnesses only comfort the doctors and impress the relatives: labels set in motion a process of causal attribution, and trigger sets of beliefs people eagerly make use upon confrontations with mental distress.

In research and clinical practice, professionals often think of diagnostic categories as realities, which create the so-called epistemic prison in the mind (Hyman 2010, p. 157): professionals think of psychological disorders as if they were discrete entities, thus obfuscating overarching and often obvious contextual influences. Disorders are seen as realities that need to be treated, or as observable surface phenomena that correspond with specific neurobiological disturbances. Research meanwhile teaches us that it is most unlikely that corresponding neurobiological patterns will ever be found for the numerous discrete disorder categories outlined in the DSM. For example, genetic studies demonstrate that no single gene variant, genomic locus, or mutation is strictly linked to any of the common mental disorders, and that particular genetic variants are often found across different disorders (Hyman 2010). Nevertheless, many professionals seem to believe that yet hidden disorder-related entities (genes, brain-related components), which are presumed to give rise to disorder-specific characteristics, do in fact exist. Such reifying belief bears witness to a cognitive bias called genetic essentialism or neuroessentialism (Dar-Nimrod and Heine 2011; Haslam 2011). Such bias narrows clinicians' and researchers' minds: "Perception of the genetic foundation as a fundamental cause leads people to devalue the role of ontogenetic, environmental, or experiential factors" (Dar-Nimrod and Heine 2011, p. 802). Interesting in this context is the plea by the Dutch psychiatrist Jim Van Os (2016, p.2) to stop using the categorical schizophrenia construct, and instead start thinking of psychosis as a mixed continuum with "extreme heterogeneity, both between and within people, in psychopathology, treatment response, and outcome." The schizophrenia concept triggers diverse fixed essentialist beliefs in professionals, thus neglecting the actual heterogeneity between patients, like the idea that schizophrenia is a highly heritable chronic brain disorder with predominantly genetic risk factors. Indeed, within such view mental disorders are seen as fixed underlying entities or essences (see also Chap. 3) that give rise to problems. Evidence, by contrast, indicates that non-essential factors like the context one lives in or life history have a serious impact on the causation of schizophrenic pathology, implicating that it is a truly biopsychosocial problem (Van Os et al. 2010, 2014). Moreover, till now no single diagnostic brain marker of schizophrenia has been found.

Interestingly, without explicit reference to Foucault, detailed studies of how psychiatrists actually dialogue with patients make clear that through concrete interactions, reification indeed takes shape. Close examination of ways in which diagnosticians ask questions makes clear that they often just check the diagnostic criteria of specific DSM disorders, thus framing patient experiences as if they were discrete categories (Ziółkowska 2012). While in daily life specific experiences have a process-like character, and are embedded in broader sets of mental representations, life histories, and interactional contexts, in diagnostic contexts they are frequently treated as isolated states with an object-like character. Linguistically this is expressed in the use of nouns instead of verbs when questioning experiences ("*Sleep* is like what?"; "are there *thoughts* about death" see: Ziółkowska 2012, p. 298). Along this way patients are constructed as passive recipients of experiences, who, from a meta-perspective, should observe disorder traits within themselves, and are invited to identify with these. This installs reification: individuals are invited to think of symptoms and disorders as discrete entities. What thus remains unacknowledged is how specific experiences, like frequent lingering on the issue of death, always take shape in idiosyncratic ways, which cannot simply be generalized from one individual to the other.

This brings us to the serious problem of laypersons embracing psy-language and adopting diagnoses in themselves or applying them to others. Even more so than professionals, laypersons tend to think of psychiatric disorders as medical diseases with known etiology or pathophysiology (Hyman 2010, p. 156). By ascribing to the language of DSM diagnoses, they too materialize diagnoses into fixed essentialist conditions thought to govern the body and/or mind. Such attributions engender stigma and blind everybody from developmental, socio-cultural and idiosyncratic interpretative factors that may be associated with a given condition; the net result is unsurprising—instead of facilitating therapeutic progress, the diagnosis itself actually might hinder change (Batstra and Thoutenhoofd 2012; Ben-Zeev et al. 2010; Mukolo et al. 2010).

Yet, in Foucault's view, reification not only creates an epistemic problem, it above all installs *power-related regimes*, thus creating social relations in which the patient gets stigmatized. In his 1973–1974 lectures at the Collège de France, he returned to the issue of psychiatric power and sharpened some of his former criticisms.[8] There he specified that power mechanisms at work in psychiatry are far from obvious, but, on the contrary, are quite subtle in character: "disciplinary power is a discrete, distributed power; it is a power which functions through networks and the visibility of which is only found in the obedience and submission of those on whom it is silently exercised" (Foucault 1973–1974, p. 22). The kind of power that Foucault points to is not personal, but relational: it is a force embedded in the doctor-patient relationship.

Detailed conversation analytic studies make clear that moral power over patient experiences are usually installed in most subtle ways (Bergmann 1992). When questioning patients diagnosticians usually apply specific rhetorical strategies. Often they refer to the uncertain

---

[8] As the transcriptions were only published in French in 2003 and in English in 2006 the historical impact of these lectures was obviously more limited than the impact of his 1965 book.

status of their knowledge (e.g., "the nurse told me that you wanted to commit suicide"), allude to experiences by referring to the opposite ("it seems that you don't feel so well"), or use mitigators and euphemistic descriptions when referring to distress ("you are kind of irritated a bit today"). This way of speaking invites patients to confess and disclose, and protects professionals from being perceived as too direct or intrusive. On the one hand such language use might be seen as considerate and affiliating in nature: the patient is invited to engage in a helping dialogue. On the other hand, as Bergmann (1992) makes clear, such speech might also be seen as a discreet intrusion in the patient's private sphere. In a subtle manner the diagnostician sets the agenda, pointing to behaviors that are seen as deviant, and thus engaging the patient to tell about personal events she perhaps didn't want to talk about. Along this way morality enters the dialogue: the patient is asked to report about what is "bad" in her life. While some patients will experience such questioning as helping and inviting, others will see it as a subtle exercise of power, against which they protest, for example, by an explicit non-collaborative attitude, or through oppositional actions.

Indeed, psychiatric diagnosis is only one way in which power manifests, and in Foucault's view the exercise of power in diagnosis is mediated by a search for truth. When an individual receives a diagnosis, he enters a so-called regime of truth: by being labeled in terms of a nosological classification system, the individual receives a definition of "who he is," or "what he has." The diagnosis provides a name for what a given individual is living through in terms of a hidden disease-thing or -process, and it invites the individual to acknowledge what the doctor proclaims. Since psychiatric diagnosis is given in the name of truth, truth that resides in psychiatric expertise, the patient is subject to the discourse of the psy-professional. It pins the individual down to an "administrative identity in which one must recognize oneself" (Foucault 1973–1974, p. 161). Thus considered, psychiatric diagnosis has an alienating effect: a diagnosis is made up of bits of psychiatric knowledge that are imposed upon an individual from without. For example, when an individual believes that he suffers from "ADHD," as indicated by his doctor, *alienation* is at play: alien criteria dictate what is going on with this person, and bring about conclusions as to whether he has a disorder or not. As the criteria used for making the diagnosis are believed to match how the individual feels and behaves, these criteria obtain a status of truth.

Foucault's historical critique came in an age where diagnosis was already under fire. He suggested that underlying the noble ethos of psychiatry, that is, curing and taking care of the mentally ill, power mechanisms and strategies of social re-adaptation were silently at work. In his view, the medicalized gaze of the physician is nothing but a pastiche that conceals the true penchant for discipline and social normalization, and this permeates the psychiatric discourse. As I will further explain in this chapter, the neo-Kraepelinian restoration movement of the 1970s consisted of a loud reconfirmation of the importance of the medical model for understanding psychopathology. Rather than addressing the fundaments of Foucault's criticisms, contemporary biomedicalization (Schomerus et al. 2012) appears to have relegated these criticisms as irrelevant. As a consequence, important questions, including the question of how psychiatric diagnosis is influenced by shifting social norms, what this shift might tell us about the nature of diagnosis, or the question of the impact diagnosis has on an individual's subjective beliefs, have remained largely unaddressed. Nonetheless, it is quite obvious that the act of characterizing individuals by means of psychiatric terminology triggers a network of beliefs and societal practices; the latter is inevitable when a discourse becomes dominant and is simply taken for granted. In other words, the discourse diagnosed individuals are imbedded in determine the way in which they are evaluated by others, as well as how they look at themselves. For example, meta-analytic research shows that biomedical explanations of mental disorders usually reduce feelings of blame and responsibility about having psychological problems, but also significantly increase pessimism about the prognosis of a disorder, and nourish the belief that individuals with mental health problems are unpredictable and dangerous (Angermeyer et al. 2011; Kvaale et al. 2013). Indeed, contrary to what many expected, biological accounts of mental disorder don't reduce prejudice and stigma toward psychiatric patients, but rather are associated with rejection: essentialist thinking about mental health problems "deepens social divides, making differences appear large, unbridgeable, inevitable, unchangeable, and ordained by nature" and "promotes division, segregation, and separation" (Haslam

2011, p. 819). Biogenetic accounts of mental disorders may be effective in reducing stigma in individuals who already have an accepting attitude toward mental health patients, but have far less effect—or even increase stigma—among individuals that hold already negative prejudice (Kvaale and Haslam 2016).

While it makes no doubt that psychiatric labels and reification might engender stigma, some traditional illness categories started functioning as *identity categories* as well, which opens up possibilities for emancipation from dominant power dynamics in society. Perhaps the best-known example is homosexuality. In the context of Western society homosexuality was long seen as a psychiatric condition, but since the 1970s it progressively got accepted as just a variety of sexual orientation. The gradual acceptance of gay marriage, which was first legally recognized in 2001 in the Netherlands, illustrates this change in attitude. Similar dynamics might now be operative for other psychiatric categories. For example, this might be the case for autism. Many autism advocates make the plea that their particular way of functioning should not be seen as indicative of disease, for which a cure or prevention strategies need to be invented, but as just a variant of human functioning, which has particular strengths and weaknesses (e.g., Grandin 2013). Guided by the idea of neurodiversity it is often indicated that autism implies certain disabilities when individuals are required to interact, which is why support is often needed, yet, it is not a malfunctioning biological condition that needs to be healed. As the self-advocacy group Aspies for Freedom formulate on their blog: "To 'cure' someone of autism would be to take away the person they are, and to replace them with someone else."[9] As a matter of fact, in his book *Far from the Tree* Andrew Solomon (2012) convincingly documents that suggestions for therapies often come across as indicative of how people without autism fail to accept peculiarities of their neighbors with autism. Self-advocacy groups like Aspies for Freedom or the Autistic Self Advocacy Network actively resist such depreciations, and want their disabilities and differences to get respected. Active identification with autism as an identity category might indeed help in getting differences respected, and in fighting prejudice. Yet, a major risk

---

[9] https://aspiesforfreedom.wordpress.com; retrieved March 15, 2016.

involved is stereotyping, whereby, just like is often the case with other minority groups, polarized ideas about autism make up a narrow perspective starting from which outsiders interpret most aspects of how an individual with autism functions. Such stereotyping might be especially problematic in people who are not actively involved with individuals with autism.

Taking into account Foucault's criticism requires an open-minded critical evaluation of how, beyond any explicit wish to exercise control, power infiltrates ordinary well-intended relationships with people with mental health problems. After all, power enters care-giving practices through the very discourse one uses. In a study of Foucault's concept of psychiatric power, Valerie Harwood (2010) argues that diagnostic labeling tends to create what she calls a *mobile asylum*: a setting in which one is locked up but that, above all, exists in the minds of those involved. While researching attention deficit hyperactivity disorder (ADHD) among children living in disadvantaged neighborhoods, Harwood (2010) observed that out of well-intended concerns, professionals tend to hastily diagnose children in crises. These diagnoses draw the attention away from difficulties they experience in their practical living contexts, that is, the family, the neighborhood, or school. Diagnoses function as truth-claims that focus on the individual, guide myriad decisions, and mobilize coercive mechanisms, which ultimately have a profound impact on the child's development. Thus considered diagnostic labeling catches the child in a series of verdicts from which they have no possible escape. In order to deal with such a mobile asylum, the potentially negative effects of diagnosis should be studied in greater detail: "to argue for the mobile asylum is to argue for the need to be alert for and recognise power and the frightening effects that certain practices, regardless of their intent, can engender" (Harwood 2010, p. 448). However, addressing implicit power dynamics requires explicit reflection on the implicit assumptions that guide diagnosis, as well as on the social interests that influence diagnostic practices. Strict belief in certain models of the mind hinder such reflection as it impedes questioning of that which seems self-evident.

Another more recent elaboration of Foucault's point of departure can be found in the works of Nikolas Rose (1996, 1999). Rose (1999, p. 7) critically appraised how psychological diagnoses and tests provide "a mechanism for rendering subjectivity into thought as a calculable force." In his view, psychological assessment and evaluation practices provide a technology, starting from which contemporary man inspects and perfects him*self*, and likewise scrutinizes and manages the *selves* of others. Through the lens of psychology, we began to think of ourselves as manageable machinery. Tests and assessments map individual differences, appraise them in terms of statistical or other social norms, and engender "techniques for the disciplining of human difference" (Rose 1996, p. 19). With reference to Gilles Deleuze, Rose argues that psychological technologies created a "fold in the soul." Indeed, by applying psychological technologies we made a problem of our own inner life: "The fold indicates a relation without an essential interior, one in which what is 'inside' is merely an infolding of an exterior" (Rose 1996, p. 37). Within this view the psy-disciplines did not so much get hold of the "essence" of psychological life, which they (as would-be natural sciences) would like to catch, but merely installed a discourse through which we attempt to predict, adapt, and govern the self. This trend toward self-government is directed by social ideals with which the individual identifies and takes as his ideal-ego. In our contemporary neo-liberal society, success, in all its varieties (beauty, performance, health, etc.), is the ideal against which the individual is measured; it is the objective in line with which the individual refines his own functioning, and in line with which he is managed by others: "In the new domain of consumption, individuals will *want* to be healthy, experts will instruct them on how to be so, and entrepreneurs will exploit and enhance this market for health" (Rose 1996, p. 162).

Indeed, researchers like Maurice Temerlin, Paul Meehl, David Rosenhan, and Robert Spitzer, and critical academics, like Thomas Szasz or Michel Foucault, arguably challenged psychiatric practice at its very core. Through their criticism, a number of fundamental problems were highlighted and research in psychopathology had to deal with these problems (i.e., the issue of reification in diagnosis; the neglect of process-thinking when diagnoses are seen as real-life entities; the naivety of having diagnoses function as lenses through which all behaviors are seen; the issue of power in well-intended care relations; and finally, the stigma that spawns in every direction from so-called diagnostic truth-claims). However, while explicit critiques of diagnostic unreliability strongly guided the revisions that led to the criterion-based DSM diagnosis, evaluations made by critical scholars in psychiatry have largely been ignored. Indeed, in the past decades many psychiatric researchers appear to have a minimal interest in the problems that critical researchers have consistently brought to the fore. As a result, the problems outlined remain as challenging as ever before.

Commotion in Psychiatry, Part III: Deinstitutionalization, Rationalization, Medicalization, and Fuzzy Decision-Making

A third motive for the switch to a criterion-based model of diagnosis (instead of a prototype-based approach) can be found in multiple changes in US society. In the 1960s and 1970s, mental health became an important topic for diverse stakeholders. Overall it was observed that during these years the need for mental health care increased dramatically.

Between 1955 and 1971 the number of patients applying for treatment doubled: in 1955 an average of slightly over 1 in 100 of all people had had a treatment episode, while in 1971 the ratio was almost 2 in 100 (Strand 2011). Despite strong investment in community mental health care and in deinstitutionalization (Grob 1987), more patients than ever before stayed in psychiatric institutions. This influx of patients meant that traditional long-term treatments could no longer be offered to everybody, which inevitably gave rise to public discontent with regard to common treatment methods. Gradually, psychotropic medication became the treatment of choice (Strand 2011; Decker 2013). In the context of the pressure put on the mental health care system, checklist-based thinking was promising. It assured a break with tradition, and it offered a transparent model for characterizing mental illness, which could then be applied to the masses in a relatively short time span.

While third parties, like the pharmaceutical industry and private and public insurers, didn't actively contribute to the creation of DSM-III, they certainly welcomed the system with open arms, as it capitalized on many of their interests and concerns (Strand 2011). With the overall increase in the number of individuals applying for treatment, financial pressures increased and psychiatric care became an activity that administrators wanted to manage following the management model of industrial companies. Insurance agencies, suspicious of long-term psychotherapeutic treatments, were increasingly interested in a rationalization of mental health care. For them a straightforward criterion-based classification system, which would also facilitate research on more effective treatments, was most promising.

The pharmaceutical industry in its turn, which by then fully endorsed the practice of randomized controlled trials, approved the criterion-based approach because of its use of explicit inclusion and exclusion criteria (Healy 2008; Strand 2011). This allowed them to delineate specific disorder groups that could be linked to specific pharmaceuticals. Such an approach was promising, not only because it fuelled the hope that pharmacological interventions could be linked with specific disorders, but above all because it enabled the marketing of specific products for specific target groups. By 2004 the industry was spending approximately twice as much per year on marketing (US$57.5 billion) than on research (US$31.5 billion) (Gagnon and Lexchin 2008).

Indeed, as Strand (2011) indicates, this exploitation of the DSM by the pharmaceutical industry, which can certainly be observed nowadays, only took off following the publication of DSM-III. An unfortunate side effect of the DSM-III is that it gave rise to *disease mongering* in psychiatry, that is, the redefinition of common discontent in psychiatric terminology: "Pharmaceutical companies are actively involved in sponsoring the definition of diseases and promoting them to both prescribers and consumers. The social construction of illness is being replaced by the corporate construction of disease" (Moynihan et al. 2002). Disease mongering has been documented for several conditions that are included in the DSM, including shyness/social phobia (Lane 2008; Moynihan et al. 2002); discontent/depression (Dehue 2008; Dowrick 2009); and inattentive behavior/ADHD (Philips 2006; Timimi and Leo 2009). Disease mongering not only generates medical consumption, but also undermines the validity of diagnostic categories: if both common misery and severe mental distress are lumped under the same label, the precise meaning of the diagnostic category ultimately becomes even more ambiguous.

While in the past three decades the pharmaceutical industry appears to have had special interest in the DSM, Allen Frances (2013), the chair of the task force that designed DSM-IV, indicates that the industry has had no direct influence on the panel for the DSM-IV. The author claims that while financial conflicts of interest have not compromised their decisions, the carefully considered decisions were certainly later exploited: "The drug industry played no role whatever in how *DSM-IV* was written, but played a deciding role in how it was misused" (Frances 2013, p. 76). Indeed, he suggests that individual experts' fads and fancies perhaps informed decisions that were made, but he does not connect these personal whims to any kind of influence made by the pharmaceutical industry. It could nevertheless be argued that there was a clear impact at that level. The pharmaceutical industry and academics studying pharmaceuticals frequently collaborate. This no doubt gives rise to loyalty, which influences decision-making. For example, Lisa Cosgrove et al. (2006) studied "conflicts of interest" in panel members of the DSM-IV and concluded that out of 170 associates, 56 % had important financial connections with the pharmaceutical industry, among which were those focusing on "mood disorders" and "schizophrenia and other psychotic disorders," which comprise the most frequently used diagnostic categories. In the panel working on the DSM-5 these conflicts of interest were even stronger: overall, 69 % of the 141 members had important financial connections with the pharmaceutical industry, reflecting a relative increase of 21 % compared to the DSM-IV panel members with such ties (Cosgrove and Krimsky 2012). More specifically, financial conflicts of interest of DSM panel members responsible for some new diagnoses in the DSM-5 (like the elimination of the bereavement exclusion criterion in major depressive disorder, binge eating disorder, and disruptive mood dysregulation disorder) and principal investigators of clinical trials for related drug treatments could be identified (Cosgrove et al. 2014). These financial ties certainly don't prove that panel members were biased. Yet considering these sponsoring connections, it is not groundless to harbor at least a degree of skepticism about the scientific independence of DSM panel members.

If task forces working on diagnostic systems want to avoid discussions about the influence of the pharmaceutical industry, they simply have to be more careful in their selection of board members, and follow a policy that assures their independence. Moreover, they should be open about the decision-making processes that lead to endorsing or changing diagnostic categories. If commercial interests do not influence the choices made by panel members, minutes of panel meetings, and open communication by diverse panel members on the decision-making processes, would offer evidence of their neutrality. Such transparency was lacking more than ever before in the development of DSM-5. In fact, panel members had to sign agreements in which they guaranteed secrecy about all meetings. This goes against the kind of transparency that is crucial to scientific practice (Peerenboom 2002), something that the former DSM-III chair Robert Spitzer too believed: "When I first heard about this agreement, I just went bonkers. Transparency is necessary if the document is to have credibility, and, in time, you're going to have people complaining all over the place that they didn't have the opportunity to challenge anything" (Spitzer, in Carey 2008). If independent peers cannot assess the methods and arguments used in obtaining a result, the truthfulness of the final result is not only suspect, it is simply insupportable.

Contra this criticism it could be argued that between 2010 and 2012 three drafts of the DSM-5 were presented online for the general public, and that the task force requested feedback each time. In other words, by setting up an online feedback platform, for the first time in the history of the DSM, the DSM-5 permitted wide-ranging input from the general public throughout its development. The DSM-5 (p. 8) states, "These three iterations of external review produced more than 13,000 individually signed comments on the website that were received and reviewed by the work groups." However, this promising development was somewhat undermined by the fact that it was (and remains) unclear as to how these comments were reviewed or analyzed, and, moreover, whether they were considered at all during the process of internal discussions and final decision-making. The same is true for commentaries endorsed by "thousands of organized petition signers" (DSM-5, p. 8). As preliminary versions of the DSM-5 were presented online, several professional societies, as well as patient and advocacy groups, submitted widely signed petitions. For example, the British Psychological Society publicly criticized the inclusion of two new diagnostic categories in the preliminary version of DSM-5: disruptive mood dysregulation disorder and attenuated psychosis syndrome. Both categories were based on vague criteria and had the potential to promulgate waves of false-positive diagnoses. The vice-president of the DSM-5 task force (Darrel Regier in *The Psychologist* 2011) responded to this criticism with a message that was simultaneously polemical and vague, using imputation (e.g., pointing to the British Psychological Society's reference to Joanna Moncrief, who endorsed ideas of Thomas Szasz) but no evidence or precise arguments that could substantiate the new categories. In the end, disruptive mood dysregulation disorder was retained as a new disorder category in the DSM-5; attenuated psychosis syndrome was cast as a disorder category for which future research is needed. Aside from the question as to whether including these diagnostic categories is acceptable, it is certainly unacceptable that the so-called evidence-based method to which decisions in DSM committees and workgroups adhere is not openly available to the scientific community.

Neo-Kraepelinian Restoration

As discussed in the previous three sections, psychiatric diagnosis was strongly under fire in the 1960s and 1970s: academic researchers revealed that its reliability and validity was insufficient, critical scholars exposed the subtle yet dark power dynamics underlying the diagnostic process and questioned the medical status of the discipline, and societal changes challenged treatment practices overall. These challenges harmed the psychiatric establishment, which was then largely populated by psychoanalytic psychiatrists. However, American psychoanalysts, who were incidentally criticized for their mediocre conventionalism by their European colleague Jacques Lacan (1953–1954, 1954–1955), could not deal very well with the challenges they were facing (Decker 2013). The overall effect was a steep decline in their influence on mental health care.

Young researchers with a renewed interest in biological psychiatry, by contrast, found an opportunity in this crisis and suggested reorganizing psychiatry along different principles. Particularly influential in this context were a group of psychiatrists affiliated with the Department of Psychiatry at Washington University in St. Louis. Their alternative approach consisted of reaffirming the *biomedical approach* to psychiatric disorders, endorsing its scientific status by embracing statistical methods and making a plea for biological research. Fundamental to this movement were the works of John Feighner, Samuel Guze, Eli Robins, and George Winokur (Decker 1997, 2013; Strand 2011). In the 1960s and early 1970s these authors promoted the idea that modern psychiatry should adopt Emil Kraepelin's descriptive approach, hence their identification as "neo-Kraepelinians" by Klerman (1978, p. 104). They condemned psychoanalysis, argued that only research with a strong focus on biology could hold any promise for psychiatry, and, more generally, aimed to refute all psychological approaches to mental suffering.

Kraepelin was attractive to them because of his classificatory focus and his assumption that mental diseases have biological causes. Like a Linnaean botanist, Kraepelin concentrated on the *form* and *essence* of cases of mental disease, as well as their various presentations, and how they change over time (Berrios and Hauser 1988; Compton and Guze 1995). By describing the symptoms presented, their onset, course, outcome, prevalence, as well as predisposing factors, familial illness history, and risk factors, he aimed to detect disease-specific biological abnormalities. Kraepelin assumed that psychiatric conditions are syndromes that make up illness entities with a biological basis and origin: "Judging from our experience in internal medicine it is a fair assumption that similar disease processes will produce identical symptom pictures, identical pathological anatomy, and identical etiology" (Kraepelin 1907, p. 117). At first Kraepelin (1907, p. 115) believed he would discover these biological abnormalities: "The principle requisite in the knowledge of mental diseases is an accurate definition of the separate disease process. In the solution of this problem one must have, on the one hand, knowledge of the physical changes in the cerebral cortex, and on the other of the mental symptoms associated with them." However, as his work progressed he postponed this dream, opting to instead develop a differentiation between psychiatric conditions by means of their associated prognosis. In his later work, Kraepelin grew more cautious of the idea of categorical differences between different disorders. While a large part of his work initially built on the distinction between dementia praecox and manic-depressive insanity, he later acknowledged a certain overlap between these conditions and entertained the possibility that they in fact reflect a unitary form of psychosis (Berrios and Hauser 1988).

The *first* idea that the neo-Kraepelinian psychiatrists put forward was that psychiatric discourse should be more strictly attuned to biomedical thinking. This implies that "concepts, strategies, and jargon of general medicine are applied to psychiatric disorders: diagnosis, differential diagnosis, etiology, pathogenesis, treatment, natural history, epidemiology, complications, and so on" (Guze 1992, p. 4). As indicated above, critical scholars like Foucault and Szasz had questioned the biomedical status of psychiatry. Along this way, they not only became archenemies of the establishment, but also seem to have provoked a reactionary move away from psychosocial lines of reasoning. The neo-Kraepelinians, who made up half of the DSM-III task force (Decker 2013, p. 98), were explicit in their wish to attune psychiatry to other medical disciplines, such as neurology. They thus revived the anatomo-clinical ideal of the nineteenth-century alienists, who aimed to connect clinically observable symptoms with anatomical lesions. Robert Spitzer, in his turn, was more subtle in his position. In the DSM-III he advocated an atheoretical position, which I discuss in Chap. 3, but nevertheless adopted many ideas from his biomedically inspired collaborators. In a later interview he suggested that, with the help of the DSM-III, psychiatry "*looked* more like a medical specialty" (Spitzer 2000, in Strand 2011, p. 300, my italics). In fact this is an interesting remark, as it leaves us wondering whether, in his opinion, it actually *is* a truly biomedical specialty.

The *second* idea that the neo-Kraepelinian psychiatrists promoted is that any further examination of mental disorders should start from "the primary organ of psychiatric illness" (Compton and Guze 1995, p. 200), that is, the brain. Indeed, in their view mental disorders are above all rooted in disorder-specific biological factors, and these make up the real substance of which symptoms, complaints, and behaviors are the observable form. Hence Compton and Guze's (1995, p. 200) statement: "the medical model is without a priori theory, but does consider brain mechanisms to be a priority." In making such a claim the authors act as though formulating priorities for one's study of psychopathology is atheoretical. Yet any choice for a particular perspective in the study of a particular phenomenon obviously reflects a theoretical preference. By prioritizing the brain, and leaving aside aspects like socio-cultural context and life events (e.g., Van Os et al. 2010), which later proved to have a serious impact on severe mental disorders, a particular theoretical choice comes to the fore.

The *third* idea that the neo-Kraepelinian psychiatrists put forward was that diagnosis in psychiatry comes down to detecting psychiatric conditions by classifying symptoms, complaints, and behaviors based on pre-established criteria (Feighner et al. 1972; Welner et al. 1974). This brought them to make the now famous statement, which is often taken for granted, that "classification *is* diagnosis" (Robins and Guze 1970, p. 983, my italics). In their view, diagnosis is not concerned with the patient qua person but with the disorder a person is carrying. The underlying idea is that disorders can be studied independently of the particularities of people's lives and thus merely require correct classification in terms of established lists of possibly occurring conditions (Klerman 1978). For them the field of psychiatry is presumed to be made up of discrete disorders that can be distinguished from one another based on five criteria: (1) clinical descriptions of symptoms that usually connect to a disorder; (2) differential diagnostic criteria that distinguish a given disorder from other conditions; (3) biomedical laboratory studies; (4) follow-up studies on the course and outcome of a disorder; (5) family studies for detecting patterns of heredity (Robins and Guze 1970; Feighner et al. 1972). The first two features make up the directly observable side of a disorder, and should, if clearly described, lead to a reliable classification of patients. The latter three components aim at detecting differences at the level of etiology and underlying pathophysiological illness mechanisms that can further explain the differences between disorders. Obviously, in their interpretation of Kraepelin, the neo-Kraepelinians focused on his early work, and assumed that neurobiological invariants could be found at the basis of observable symptoms. Along this way, Kraepelin's later evolutions, which questioned categorical distinctions between disorders, were neglected. As already indicated, Spitzer strongly believed in these classificatory principles and assumed that this approach would enhance diagnostic reliability (Spitzer and Fleiss 1974). He consequently used them as a basis for elaborating the DSM-III disorder categories.

In the first paper that actually introduced the format of criterion-based diagnosis, Feighner et al. (1972) came to describe 16 disorders that cohered reasonably well with the five basic principles that should be fulfilled for each discrete category. Among others, these included schizophrenia, hysteria, obsessional neurosis, primary affective disorders (depression and mania), as well the then controversial category of homosexuality. All were considered to be reasonably valid diagnostic categories. In 1974 R.A. Woodruff and colleagues reduced this list to 12, and in 1978 Spitzer, Endicot, and Robins extended it again to 25 by elaborating the differentiation between *forms* of affective disorder (see Table 2.3). Indeed in 1978, only two years before the publication of DSM-III, Spitzer and colleagues published their *Research Diagnostic Criteria* (RDC), which aimed at enhancing reliability by providing standardized sets of factors that had to be evaluated. They tested these operationally defined disorder categories in three small-scale studies, using judges that were highly familiar with the RDC. One of these studies, including 60 patients, used a test-retest design: in a timeframe of two days two psychiatrists evaluated the same patient using a standardized interview schedule. The authors presented their observed kappa values as a scientific achievement: "The results of these three studies indicate that the reliability of the RDC categories is *very high*" (Spitzer et al. 1978, p. 779, my italics). Remarkably, in contrast to their earlier study, Spitzer and colleagues didn't define the norms upon which they based the evaluation of their kappa values and as a consequence it is unclear how they came to the conclusion that the reliability of these diagnostic categories is "very high." This might indicate that Spitzer and his associates were actually very selective in how they used the kappa statistic. If they had used the norms Spitzer used with Fleiss (1974), they would have concluded that out of the 18 conditions tested, 2 have a high reliability; 12 have satisfactory reliability, and 4 have unacceptable reliability (see Table 2.3). Indeed, it seems Spitzer and associates changed their standards in terms of the conclusions they wanted to draw. Even based on the norms of Landis and Koch (1977) or those used by Clarke et al. (2013) the assertion of "very

Table 2.3 Kappa coefficients for research diagnostic criteria disorders adapted from Spitzer et al. (1978, p. 779), and three sets of interpretations of the kappa coefficient using different norms

Disorder category	Kappa	Interpretation Spitzer and Fleiss (1974) norms	Interpretation Landis and Koch (1977) norms	Interpretation Clarke et al. (2013) norms
PEO Schizophrenia	0.65	Unacceptable	Fair to good	Very good
PEO Schizoaffective disorder Manic type	0.79	Satisfactory	Excellent	Very good
PEO Schizoaffective disorder Depressed type	0.73	Satisfactory	Fair to good	Very good
PEO Manic disorder	0.82	Satisfactory	Excellent	Excellent
PEO Major depressive disorder	0.90	Satisfactory	Excellent	Excellent
PEO Alcoholism	1.0	High	Excellent	Excellent
PEO Drug abuse	0.92	High	Excellent	Excellent
LD schizophrenia	0.73	Satisfactory	Fair to good	Very good
LD Schizoaffective disorder Depressed type	0.70	Satisfactory	Fair to good	Very good
LD Manic disorder	0.77	Satisfactory	Excellent	Very good
LD Hypomanic disorder	0.56	Unacceptable	Fair to good	Good
LD Major depressive disorder	0.71	Satisfactory	Fair to good	Very good
LD Alcoholism	0.95	Satisfactory	Excellent	Excellent
LD Drug abuse	0.73	Satisfactory	Fair to good	Very good
LD Labile personality	0.70	Satisfactory	Fair to good	Very good
LD Bipolar I	0.40	Unacceptable	Fair to good	Moderate
LD Recurrent unipolar	0.80	Satisfactory	Excellent	Excellent
LD Intermittent depressive Disorder	0.57	Unacceptable	Fair to good	Good

PEO present episode only, *LD* lifetime diagnosis

high" reliability is clearly an overestimation. Such biased use of evaluation standards sheds doubt on the scientific integrity of the DSM-III architects. Above all, they seem to have been marketing a biomedical approach in psychiatry, which they disguised by presenting quantitative output that they interpreted in a partial way. Moreover, given the fact that those who tested the RDC were also those who developed them (adding to that the small sample used in the study), drawing such firm conclusions is unjustifiable (Decker 2013).

Compared to the DSM-II (1968), which counted 182 disorders, the lists of presumably valid diagnoses presented by Feighner et al. (1972), Woodruff et al. (1974), and Spitzer et al. (1978) were much smaller. Their trimmed lists of 16, 12, and 25 categories might respectively indicate that an age of new austerity was needed. Yet, this is not what happened. Despite its scientific aspirations the DSM-III was far less parsimonious than any system before, in terms of the 265 illness categories it discerned. Nonetheless, it was presumed that these categories reflected discrete disorders. Spitzer clearly relaxed the requirements that the neo-Kraepelinians had formulated for valid diagnostic categories: concentrating on symptomatic description alone, the DSM-III set aside the principle that diagnostic categories had to be based on biomedical laboratory studies, follow-up studies, and patterns of heredity (Robins and Guze 1970; Feighner et al. 1972).

In this context, Spitzer seemed to be using a double standard: while he believed that in research settings the number of diagnostic categories had to be limited in order to avoid false-positive diagnosis, he also argued that in clinical contexts, an extensive list of disorders with flexible criteria was needed in order to avoid false-negative diagnosis (Decker 2013, pp. 176–177). By making this choice, it looks like he wanted to boost diagnostic reliability in scientific studies, thus promoting the credibility of his approach. In clinical practice, by contrast, diagnosticians using the DSM-III had and still have to make choices based on far more elaborate lists of disorders, which increases the possibility that different diagnosticians use different labels to name the same problem. More recent naturalistic diagnostic research illustrates this problem. For example, in a study focusing on conduct disorder Kirk and Hsieh (2004) created a vignette with a short description of a 12-year-old boy.

The vignette was attuned to the diagnostic criteria of conduct disorder, as defined in the DSM-IV. Starting from this short description of the boy, a sample of 1334 psychiatrists, psychologists, and social workers with broad experience working with young adults (with an average age of 20.7 years) were asked to give him a DSM diagnosis. The group differed substantially in their diagnoses: 29 DSM clinical disorders were proposed as the primary diagnosis and only 45.5 % actually diagnosed conduct disorder, thus demonstrating that consistency in diagnosis is weak. Further examination of the data set demonstrated that brief descriptors of the boy's ethnic background influenced the diagnosis significantly and that diagnosticians gave significantly different diagnoses based on their professional specialty and years of experience (Pottick et al. 2007). More fundamentally, clinicians' assumptions about the presence of an internal dysfunction strongly determined the diagnostic choices they made (Kirk and Hsieh 2009). This shows that the interpretation of mental symptoms is not as strongly based on the descriptive features that diagnostic criteria supposedly capture, as people often believe.

Moreover, as the number of categories increased substantially in the DSM-III, it became increasingly unlikely that the plethora of new disorder categories, all created in the workgroup discussions (Decker 2013), would ultimately prove to be valid. Nonetheless, they were avidly used in clinical practice. Irrespective of relatively minor changes, these categories are also included in the DSM-5. Nevertheless, the DSM-5 differs substantially from the DSM-III and DSM-IV in terms of its basic assumptions concerning the disorder categories. Whereas the DSM-III and DSM-IV presumed that disorder categories are discrete, this is no longer the case in DSM-5 (Regier et al. 2013). Given the frequently observed comorbidity between different DSM conditions and the fact that biomedical studies fail to support the idea that DSM disorders correspond with delineated biological conditions, the DSM-5 committee gave up on the idea of discrete disorders (Hyman 2010). It is quite paradoxical, however, that the DSM-5 nevertheless holds on to the diagnostic categories defined by its predecessors.

Diagnostic Reliability Since the DSM-III

We started this chapter with the observation that the DSM is often praised for its reliability: The DSM-III and its successors are often presumed to be much more reliable than earlier diagnostic systems. However, the question as to what evidence substantiates such a belief remains open. In this section I review this presumption, focusing on key reliability studies concerning the DSM-III as well as subsequent editions of the manual. Given our focus on the statistical kappa coefficient the following section is quite technical. However, a careful understanding of important psychometric studies published over the past 25 years is key to evaluating the claim that *since the DSM-III great progress has been made at the level of reliability*. We will start by looking at the initial reliability study that was conducted for the DSM-III and then look more closely at the DSM-5 field trial.

As the DSM-III was being developed, Spitzer and associates (1979) examined 25 out of 265 diagnostic categories with a test-retest design in a field trial[10] (Spitzer et al. 1979). In total 131 patients were evaluated by two volunteering psychiatrists who selected participants from their work settings. This time a kappa value of 0.70 or more was considered to be "high," and indicative of "good agreement" (Spitzer et al. 1979, pp. 816–817). Importantly, the study did not evaluate the reliability of exact diagnostic categories, but examined clusters of disorders, assuming that diagnoses are identical if they belong to the same cluster. Given the fact that all DSM-III disorders were presumed to be discrete entities, the choice of only testing clusters in which disorder categories were grouped is strange. In other words, the field trial didn't actually test the disorder categories that the DSM-III offered as an answer to presumably unscientific pre-DSM-III diagnostic practices.

The results of the field trial can be found in Table 2.4. We again interpret the kappa coefficient starting from the norms formulated in Table 2.1. Spitzer and associates (1979, p. 818) concluded that for most

---

[10] In the DSM-III the results from the field trial can be found in Appendix F (pp. 467–472). Unfortunately, no distinctions were made between patients simultaneously diagnosed by the two psychiatrists or those evaluated in a test-retest design. Therefore, I cannot include these in my review.

Table 2.4 Kappa coefficients from the DSM-III field trials, adapted from Spitzer et al. (1979), and three sets of interpretations of the kappa coefficient using different norms

Disorder category	Kappa	Interpretation Spitzer and Fleiss (1974) norms	Interpretation Landis and Koch (1977) norms	Interpretation Clarke et al. (2013) norms
Disorders of infancy, childhood or adolescence	0.81	Satisfactory	Excellent	Excellent
Mental retardation	0.85	Satisfactory	Excellent	Excellent
Disorders of late adolescence	0.66	Unacceptable	Fair to good	Very good
Eating disorders	0.85	Satisfactory	Excellent	Excellent
Organic mental disorders	0.83	Satisfactory	Excellent	Excellent
Senile and pre-senile dementias	0.74	Satisfactory	Fair to good	Very good
Substance induced syndromes	0.74	Satisfactory	Fair to good	Very good
With unknown etiology	0.72	Satisfactory	Fair to good	Very good
Substance use disorders	0.74	Satisfactory	Fair to good	Very good
Schizophrenic disorders	0.82	Satisfactory	Excellent	Excellent
Paranoid disorders	1.0	High	Excellent	Excellent
Schizoaffective disorders	0.53	Unacceptable	Fair to good	Good
Affective disorders	0.59	Unacceptable	Fair to good	Good
Major affective disorders	0.65	Unacceptable	Fair to good	Very good
Chronic minor affective disorder	0.29	Unacceptable	Poor	Questionable
Psychoses not elsewhere classified	0.43	Unacceptable	Fair to good	Good
Anxiety disorders	0.43	Unacceptable	Fair to good	Good

(*continued*)

Table 2.4 (continued)

Disorder category	Kappa	Interpretation Spitzer and Fleiss (1974) norms	Interpretation Landis and Koch (1977) norms	Interpretation Clarke et al. (2013) norms
Factitious disorders	1.0	High	Excellent	Excellent
Somatoform disorders	0.66	Unacceptable	Fair to good	Very good
Dissociative disorders	0.00	Unacceptable	Poor	Unacceptable
Psychosexual disorders	1.0	High	Excellent	Excellent
Paraphilias	1.0	High	Excellent	Excellent
Psychosexual dysfunctions	1.0	High	Excellent	Excellent
Adjustment disorders	0.60	Unacceptable	Fair to good	Very good
Disorders of impulsive control	0.00	Unacceptable	Poor	Unacceptable

of the diagnoses reliability is "quite good and, in general is higher than that previously achieved using DSM-I and DSM-II." Given the fact that for 11 of the 25 categories the observed kappa is below their own standard of 0.70 this conclusion seems overly optimistic. The overall kappa coefficient they observed for Axis-I disorders (clinical syndromes) was 0.66 and for Axis-II disorders (personality disorders and specific developmental disorders) it was 0.54. Generally, the results of this study are better than those of the review study by Spitzer and Fleiss (1974), yet the small sample size used renders it impossible to make relevant comparisons. Indeed, the DSM-III field trial started from a sample that was substantially smaller than the 1726 patients Spitzer and Fleiss (1974) included in their review of pre-DSM-III diagnosis. Spitzer and his associates (1979) calculated kappa values for 25 conditions, but used only 131 patients, which implies that some of the kappa coefficients were based on a very low number of patients. Unfortunately, they didn't discuss the distribution of patients over the different conditions. As a result, the kappa coefficients that were calculated cannot be considered as good estimates.

Other test-retest reliability studies focusing on the DSM-III or the revised DSM-III (DSM-III-R[11]) that included sufficient numbers of patients per tested condition yielded mixed results. For example, a DSM-III-R test-retest reliability study in Germany that examined 5 disorder categories with 100 patients and 4 raters (Hiller et al. 1993) observed a mean kappa value of 0.53, as well as substantial differences between disorders: schizophrenia: kappa = 0.51; schizophreniform/acute and transient psychotic disorder: kappa = 0.50; schizoaffective disorder: kappa = 0.08; major depression: kappa = 0.80; bipolar disorder: kappa = 0.65.

High-quality test-retest reliability studies on the DSM-III were not performed until the *Structured Clinical Interview for DSM* (SCID) was published. This diagnostic interview was developed in order to provide a standardized assessment of DSM disorders (Spitzer et al. 1984). The use of a structured interview has a heightening effect on reliability: because questions clinicians ask are uniform and clinical improvisation is restricted, variability in patients' answers diminishes, which facilitates consistency in diagnostic classification across judges. The first edition of the SCID was developed for the DSM-III, but the version developed for the DSM-III-R was more frequently used in research. Different versions of the SCID were developed for examining various clinical syndromes (Axis I in DSM-III until DSM-IV-TR) and diagnosing personality disorders (Axis II in DSM-III until DSM-IV-TR). A version of the SCID for DSM-5 (SCID-5) is also published, but reliability studies are not yet available (First et al. 2016).

In 1992 Janet Williams and ten other collaborators, including Robert Spitzer, published a large multisite test-retest study that examined the reliability of the SCID for DSM-III-R Axis-I disorders.[12] Six clinics in the USA and one in Germany were involved. The study examined how well clinicians agree when diagnosing patients from psychiatric clinics. Next to that, they examined inter-rater agreement when testing mentally

---

[11] Compared to the DSM-III, the DSM-III-R, published in 1987, mainly contained changes in diagnostic criteria. Next to that, some DSM-III disorder categories were deleted from the DSM-III-R, while others were added. In total the DSM-III-R counts 292 diagnoses, an increase of 27 compared to the DSM-III.

[12] The SCID was tested in several other studies, sometimes yielding better results (e.g., Skre et al. 1991). Yet, typically these studies used smaller sample sizes, as a result of which estimated kappa values cannot be thought of as stable (Williams et al. 1992). Often data were collected in only one setting.

Table 2.5 Kappa coefficients from SCID-I test-retest study in psychiatric patients by Williams et al. (1992), and three sets of interpretations of the kappa coefficient using different norms

Disorder category	Kappa	Interpretation Spitzer and Fleiss (1974) norms	Interpretation Landis and Koch (1977) norms	Interpretation Clarke et al. (2013) norms
Bipolar disorder	0.84	Satisfactory	Excellent	Excellent
Major depression	0.64	Unacceptable	Fair to good	Very good
Dysthymia	0.40	Unacceptable	Fair to good	Good
Schizophrenia	0.65	Unacceptable	Fair to good	Very good
Schizophreniform disorder	0.59	Unacceptable	Fair to good	Good
Schizoaffective disorder	0.63	Unacceptable	Fair to good	Very good
Delusional disorder	0.69	Unacceptable	Fair to good	Very good
Alcohol abuse/ dependence	0.75	Satisfactory	Fair to good	Very good
Other drug abuse/ dependence	0.84	Satisfactory	Excellent	Excellent
Panic disorder	0.58	Unacceptable	Fair to good	Good
Agoraphobia	0.43	Unacceptable	Fair to good	Good
Social phobia	0.47	Unacceptable	Fair to good	Good
Simple phobia	0.52	Unacceptable	Fair to good	Good
Obsessive-compulsive disorder	0.59	Unacceptable	Fair to good	Good
Generalized anxiety disorder	0.56	Unacceptable	Fair to good	Good
Hypochondrias	0.57	Unacceptable	Fair to good	Good
Anorexia nervosa	0.72	Satisfactory	Fair to good	Very good
Bulimia nervosa	0.86	Satisfactory	Excellent	Excellent

distressed people from the general community. Twenty-five trained raters were involved and in total 390 patients and 202 non-patients were tested. Kappa coefficients were calculated for categories that were diagnosed at least ten times. Table 2.5 contains interpreted results for current[13] diagnoses in psychiatric patients. Compared to the results obtained for pre-DSM-III reliability studies (Table 2.2) these reliability coefficients are only slightly better, which is also what Kutchins and Kirk (1997) suggest

---

[13] The study also includes kappa coefficients calculated for lifetime diagnoses. For some diagnostic categories these were slightly better than those for current diagnosis.

Table 2.6 Kappa coefficients from SCID-I test-retest study in non-patients by Williams et al. (1992), and three sets of interpretations of the kappa coefficient using different norms

Disorder category	Kappa	Interpretation Spitzer and Fleiss (1974) norms	Interpretation Landis and Koch (1977) norms	Interpretation Clarke et al. (2013) norms
Major depression	0.42	Unacceptable	Fair to good	Good
Dysthymia	0.53	Unacceptable	Fair to good	Good
Panic disorder	0.59	Unacceptable	Fair to good	Good
Social phobia	0.41	Unacceptable	Fair to good	Good
Simple phobia	0.48	Unacceptable	Fair to good	Good
Adjustment disorder	0.19	Unacceptable	Poor	Unacceptable

in their critical evaluation of the DSM-III. Indeed, considered from the Spitzer and Fleiss (1974) norms, 13 categories have an unacceptable reliability, 5 have satisfactory reliability, but none is highly reliable, which is remarkable given the fact that the structured nature of the SCID should yield heightened reliability scores. The Landis and Koch (1977) norms and the norms used by Clarke and associates (2013) lead to more positive interpretations, yet only the results for mood disorders are substantially better than those obtained 20 years earlier.

The results from the non-patient group (Table 2.6), in their turn, indicate that the correspondence between raters is lower than in the clinical group. Actually, these are at the level of the reliabilities observed by Spitzer and Fleiss (1974). Considered from the Spitzer and Fleiss (1974) norms these kappa values cast doubt on the typical neo-Kraepelinian presumption (Klerman 1978) that mental disorders make up illness conditions that are clearly delineated from normal states of mind.

In a next step, these researchers also tested the inter-rater reliability of the SCID for personality disorders (First et al. 1995): on a pairwise basis, 25 trained judges evaluated 103 psychiatric patients and 181 non-clinical participants. The results (Tables 2.7 and 2.8) indicate that the kappa values are somewhat lower than for the SCID assessment of clinical disorders (Axis I). Raters disagreed substantially in the non-clinical group in particular, bringing the level of agreement below the level observed in pre-DSM-III diagnosis.

Table 2.7 Kappa coefficients from SCID-II test-retest study in psychiatric patients by First et al. (1995), and three sets of interpretations of the kappa coefficient using different norms

Personality disorder category	Kappa	Interpretation Spitzer and Fleiss (1974) norms	Interpretation Landis and Koch (1977) norms	Interpretation Clarke et al. (2013) norms
Paranoid	0.68	Unacceptable	Fair to good	Very good
Histrionic	0.74	Satisfactory	Fair to good	Very good
Narcissistic	0.43	Unacceptable	Fair to good	Good
Borderline	0.40	Unacceptable	Fair to good	Good
Anti-social	0.71	Satisfactory	Fair to good	Very good
Avoidant	0.71	Satisfactory	Fair to good	Very good
Dependent	0.42	Unacceptable	Fair to good	Good
Obsessive-compulsive	0.24	Unacceptable	Poor	Questionable
Passive-aggressive	0.59	Unacceptable	Fair to good	Good
Self-defeating	0.40	Unacceptable	Fair to good	Good

Table 2.8 Kappa coefficients from SCID-II test-retest study in non-patients by First et al. (1995), and three sets of interpretations of the kappa coefficient using different norms

Personality disorder category	Kappa	Interpretation Spitzer and Fleiss (1974) norms	Interpretation Landis and Koch (1977) norms	Interpretation Clarke et al. (2013) norms
Paranoid	0.47	Unacceptable	Fair to good	Good
Histrionic	0.51	Unacceptable	Fair to good	Good
Narcissistic	0.42	Unacceptable	Fair to good	Good
Borderline	0.57	Unacceptable	Fair to good	Good
Avoidant	0.35	Unacceptable	Poor	Questionable
Dependent	0.59	Unacceptable	Fair to good	Good
Obsessive-compulsive	0.24	Unacceptable	Poor	Questionable
Passive-aggressive	0.31	Unacceptable	Poor	Questionable
Self-defeating	0.12	Unacceptable	Poor	Unacceptable

The DSM-IV and DSM-IV-TR, published in 1994 and 2000 respectively, did not bring about major changes in the system. Overall, criteria that reflected patients' experience of distress were added; several other diagnostic criteria were altered; some disorder categories were removed while others were introduced. This resulted in a total of 297 diagnoses. The field trials that accompanied the DSM-IV didn't specifically focus on test-retest reliability. Concentrating on specific disorders, they mainly examined how changes in diagnostic criteria altered prevalence rates (e.g., Keller et al. 1996). Studies using the SCID for DSM-IV diagnoses, in their turn, yielded results that were similar to those obtained with the SCID for the DSM-III-R. For example, in a small-size multisite reliability study, Zanarini and associates (2000) evaluated 52 psychiatric cases with multiple trained judges in a test-retest design. Of the nine personality disorders tested, eight had fair to good reliability according to the Landis and Koch (1977) standard, while one (paranoid personality disorder) had poor reliability.

Notwithstanding all rhetoric on the good reliability of the DSM since 1980 it was only with the DSM-5 field trials that a major test-retest reliability study was conducted with a sample size that was comparable to the 1726 patients that Spitzer and Fleiss (1974) included in their review. The DSM-5 field trials tested the reliability of 27 diagnostic categories in adults as well as in children and adolescents (Clarke et al. 2013; Regier et al. 2013). Two hundred and eighty-six clinicians participated, and a total of 1466 adult patients and 616 pediatric patients were evaluated by 2 trained clinicians separately. Only patients with problems that were relevant in terms of the 27 tested conditions were included. The obtained kappa coefficients as well as our interpretation of these values can be found in Table 2.9 for adults and Table 2.10 for children.

Despite the claim in the introduction of the DSM-5 (p. 5) that "DSM has been the cornerstone of substantial progress in reliability," the results are simply no better than those found by Spitzer and Fleiss (1974) (Table 2.2). Of the 18 categories examined by Spitzer and Fleiss (1974), 15 had an unacceptable reliability according to their norms. Applying these norms to the DSM-5 field trial makes clear that 14 of the 15 diagnoses in adults and all seven pediatric diagnoses have an unacceptable reliability. In terms of the kappa evaluation norms formulated by Clarke et al. (2013), four pre-DSM-III categories had a very good reliability, eight a good reliability, and six a questionable reliability. In terms of these norms three categories from the DSM-5 field trial for adult patients had a very good reliability, seven a good reliability, four a questionable reliability,

Table 2.9 Kappa coefficients from the DSM-5 field trials in adult patients (Regier et al. 2013) and three sets of interpretations of the kappa coefficient using different norms

Disorder category	Kappa	Interpretation Spitzer and Fleiss (1974) norms	Interpretation Landis and Koch (1977) norms	Interpretation Clarke et al. (2013) norms
Schizophrenia	0.46	Unacceptable	Fair to good	Good
Schizoaffective disorder	0.50	Unacceptable	Fair to good	Good
Bipolar I disorder	0.56	Unacceptable	Fair to good	Good
Major depressive disorder	0.28	Unacceptable	Poor	Questionable
Mixed anxiety-depressive disorder	0.00	Unacceptable	Poor	Unacceptable
Generalized anxiety disorder	0.20	Unacceptable	Poor	Questionable
Post-traumatic stress disorder	0.67	Unacceptable	Fair to good	Very good
Complex somatic disorder	0.61	Unacceptable	Fair to good	Very good
Binge eating disorder	0.56	Unacceptable	Fair to good	Good
Alcohol use disorder	0.40	Unacceptable	Fair to good	Good
Mild neurocognitive disorder	0.48	Unacceptable	Fair to good	Good
Major neurocognitive disorder	0.78	Satisfactory	Excellent	Very good
Mild traumatic brain injury	0.36	Unacceptable	Poor	Questionable
Anti-social personality disorder	0.21	Unacceptable	Poor	Questionable
Borderline personality disorder	0.54	Unacceptable	Fair to good	Good

and one an unacceptable reliability. In the DSM-5 field trial for children, two diagnoses had a very good reliability, two a good reliability, two a questionable reliability, and two an unacceptable reliability. Whereas those categories with unacceptable reliability have been omitted from the

Table 2.10 Kappa coefficients from the DSM-5 field trials in pediatric patients (Regier et al. 2013) and three sets of interpretations of the kappa coefficient using different norms

Disorder category	Kappa	Interpretation Spitzer and Fleiss (1974) norms	Interpretation Landis and Koch (1977) norms	Interpretation Clarke et al. (2013) norms
Autism spectrum disorders	0.69	Unacceptable	Fair to good	Very good
ADHD	0.61	Unacceptable	Fair to good	Very good
Disruptive mood dysregulation	0.25	Unacceptable	Poor	Questionable
Mixed anxiety-depressive disorder	0.05	Unacceptable	Poor	Unacceptable
Major depressive disorder	0.28	Unacceptable	Poor	Questionable
Avoidant/restrictive food intake	0.48	Unacceptable	Fair to good	Good
Oppositional defiant disorder	0.40	Unacceptable	Fair to good	Good

final version of the DSM-5, it remains that the kappa values anno 2013 are comparable to those obtained anno 1974.[14]

What is more, an important problem coming to the fore in the DSM-5 field trial is that the diagnosis of mood disorders (the most frequently made psychiatric diagnosis) is no more reliable than it was found to be in the review study of Spitzer and Fleiss (1974). In the 1970s affective disorders in particular had a questionable reliability; 40 years later the reliability coefficients are even worse. This might be a result of defining depression too broadly, including diagnostic criteria that are far too vague, and neglecting context variables (Maj 2012). Contra this criticism it could be argued that throughout the years a number of standardized interviews that have a good reliability were developed for assessing depression (e.g., Trajkovic et al. 2011; Williams and Kobak 2008). Yet,

---

[14] Contra this interpretation it could be argued that across studies the statistical formulae used for estimating reliability indices are slightly different. For example, the DSM field trial took into account the population prevalence of tested conditions, while the studies from the 1970s did not. These differences have to do with the evolution of statistical methodology and the availability of accurate prevalence data. However, throughout the years the interpretation of the kappa coefficient largely remained the same, which is why comparisons can indeed be made.

these were developed apart from the DSM, and were not integrated into subsequent editions of the manual.

Interestingly, the interpretation of the DSM-5 field trials by the researching team (Regier et al. 2013) as well as by editors of the *American Journal of Psychiatry* (Freedman et al. 2013) particularly focuses on the "new blooms" the field trials produced, leaving aside some of the "old thorns" the study brought to the fore.

One problem that both interpretations acknowledge concerns the poor results for depression- and anxiety-related conditions. While these poor results are mainly attributed to comorbidity between these conditions (including major depression, generalized anxiety, alcohol use, and post-traumatic stress disorder [PTSD]), reflection on the system that produces such high comorbidity rates is yet to be made. Moreover, these interpretations (Freedman et al. 2013; Regier et al. 2013) have not mobilized any kind of shift toward putting into question the overrated claim of good diagnostic reliability since the DSM-III. A further issue that remains wholly neglected is that whereas this field trial was able to estimate reliabilities for *some* disorders, the majority of DSM-5 diagnostic categories were not tested at all: the DSM-5 counts 347[15] disorder categories, but kappa coefficients could be calculated only for 20 conditions (6 %). Moreover, of those categories only 14 had a good or very good reliability, which means that only 4 % of the DSM-5 categories have been shown to have sufficient reliability. Indeed, since the inter-rater reliability of the majority of DSM-5 categories remains untested, the idea that the DSM is a reliable instrument is simply wrong. In their DSM-5 editorial, by contrast, Freedman et al. (2013, p. 3) conclude: "For a general psychiatric practice, the diagnostic reliability data suggest that two-thirds of patients will receive a reliable DSM-5 principal diagnosis at the first visit." Given the fact that acceptable reliability coefficients have been observed for only 4 % of the DSM categories, and given the poor reliabilities observed for anxiety- and depression-related psychopathology, this claim is seriously

---

[15] This count is based on the list provided in the preface of the DSM-5 (pp. xiii–xxxiii). In line with the DSM-5's distinction between *subtypes*, which refer to "mutually exclusive and jointly exhaustive phenomenological subgroupings within a diagnosis," and *specifiers*, which "are not intended to be mutually exclusive or jointly exhaustive" (DSM-5, p. 21), we took into account subtypes, but not specifiers.

overrated. In other words, just because the field trials indicate that two out of three conditions had good kappa coefficients it does not follow that the same is true for all other DSM-5 categories (94 % of the manual). Moreover, there is no discussion of the norms used for interpreting the kappa coefficient in any publications by those responsible for the DSM-5. Compared to frequently used standards in psychiatric research (Baer and Blais 2010) the norms used in the DSM-5 field trials were exceptionally low (Frances 2012; Vanheule et al. 2014). Such use of low standards might reflect a tactical maneuver to boost bad results.

The main achievements Regier et al. (2013) and Freedman and associates focus on concern the very good reliabilities observed for a number of conditions, like PTSD in adults and ADHD in children. Considered from the norms of Clarke et al. (2013) these disorders can indeed be classified in reliable ways. However, these disorders have been contested at the level of validity. For example, in an analysis of the criteria that make up PTSD, Gerald Rosen and Scott Lilienfeld (2008) conclude "that virtually all core assumptions and hypothesized mechanisms lack compelling or consistent empirical support." Similarly, critical examinations of ADHD reveal that fundamental questions on the nature and meaning of the ADHD construct remain unanswered (Batstra and Thoutenhoofd 2012; Parens and Johnston 2011; Rafalovich 2004; Timimi and Leo 2009). Another success the authors focus on concerns their proposition that schizophrenia, bipolar disorder, and schizoaffective disorder can be distinguished reasonably well. This observation is important, but perhaps not that surprising, since the SCID already distinguishes these conditions reasonably well (Williams et al. 1992). Nevertheless, whereas the field trial underlines the differentiation between these psychosis-related conditions, research pointing to the overlap between them must not be ignored (Angst 2002; Hyman 2010; McNally 2011; Van Os 2016) as it suggests that categorical distinctions between these disorders might not be valid.

In a later reliability study, Chmielewski et al. (2015) pointed out that the disappointing kappa coefficients in the DSM-5 field trials might be an effect of the method the researchers used. Just like the studies synthesized by Spitzer and Fleiss (1974), the DSM-5 field trial used a test-retest design: two or more diagnosticians evaluate one patient, with a small time interval between the interviews. Another method for evaluating diagnostic reliability is audio- or video-recording: "In this method, one clinician conducts the interview and provides diagnoses; a second 'blinded' clinician then provides an independent set of diagnoses based on recordings of the interview" (Chmielewski 2015, p. 765). Such a method usually yields higher reliability estimates. In their study, Chmielewski and colleagues evaluated 12 DSM-IV disorders, and included 339 psychiatric patients. All were diagnosed with the test-retest method using the SCID interview for DSM-IV and a one-week interval between both interviews. For 49 patients the audio-recording method was used as well.

The obtained kappa coefficients, and interpretation of these values, can be found in Tables 2.11 and 2.12. In the test-retest condition the mean kappa was 0.47. Starting from the strict kappa evaluation standards of Spitzer and Fleiss (1974) all diagnoses have unacceptably low reliabilities (see Table 2.11). Using the norms of Clarke et al. (2013) four disorders have very good diagnostic reliability, including major depressive disorder, panic disorder, psychosis, and substance use disorder. Five conditions were diagnosed with good reliability (obsessive-compulsive disorder, PTSD, bipolar I disorder, specific phobia, generalized anxiety disorder), and three have questionable reliabilities (social phobia, dysthymic disorder, other bipolar disorders). Overall, this study yields reliability indices that are similar to those observed in the other studies we reviewed, albeit that kappa values are lower than in the study by Williams and associates (1992), which also used the standardized SCID interview. Remarkably, just like in the other SCID study (Williams et al. 1992) the diagnostic reliability of major depressive disorder and generalized anxiety disorder is much better than in the DSM-5 field trial. In the test condition where a second diagnostician used audiotaped interviews conducted by a first diagnostician, by contrast, reliability indices are much better, reaching a mean kappa value of 0.80 (see Table 2.12). Of the 12 conditions tested in the study by Chmielewski et al. (2015), 11 had excellent or very good reliabilities, as evaluated with the DSM-5 thresholds (Clarke et al. 2013).

Most remarkably, both test conditions yielded highly different results. This curious outcome indicates that perhaps the problem is not

Table 2.11 Kappa coefficients from SCID test-retest study in psychiatric patients by Chmielewski et al. (2015), and three sets of interpretations of the kappa coefficient using different norms

Disorder category	Kappa	Interpretation Spitzer and Fleiss (1974) norms	Interpretation Landis and Koch (1977) norms	Interpretation Clarke et al. (2013) norms
Obsessive-compulsive disorder	0.41	Unacceptable	Fair to good	Good
Major depressive disorder	0.60	Unacceptable	Fair to good	Very good
Social phobia	0.25	Unacceptable	Unacceptable	Questionable
Post-traumatic stress disorder	0.52	Unacceptable	Unacceptable	Good
Panic disorder	0.60	Unacceptable	Fair to good	Very good
Psychotic disorder	0.60	Unacceptable	Fair to good	Very good
Substance use disorder	0.62	Unacceptable	Fair to good	Very good
Dysthymic disorder	0.22	Unacceptable	Fair to good	Questionable
Bipolar I disorder	0.58	Unacceptable	Unacceptable	Good
Specific phobia	0.54	Unacceptable	Fair to good	Good
Other bipolar (II or NOS)	0.25	Unacceptable	Fair to good	Questionable
Generalized anxiety disorder	0.45	Unacceptable	Fair to good	Good

only a matter of diagnosticians' divergent opinions about psychological distress, and of their idiosyncratic ways of interpreting mental health symptoms. After all, the test condition with audiotapes demonstrates that when using exactly the same patient accounts, evaluators make very similar classificatory decisions. A conclusion we can draw from these results is that perhaps the accounts individuals give about mental distress are not very stable. The entire enterprise of evaluating reliability presupposes stability both at the side of diagnosticians' evaluation and at the side of the patients' account. Yet if patient accounts of distress have a different outline and character across interviews, the search for good reliability will always be disappointing unless the nature and

Table 2.12 Kappa coefficients from audio-recording reliability study in psychiatric patients by Chmielewski et al. (2015), and three sets of interpretations of the kappa coefficient using different norms

Disorder category	Kappa	Interpretation Spitzer and Fleiss (1974) norms	Interpretation Landis and Koch (1977) norms	Interpretation Clarke et al. (2013) norms
Obsessive-compulsive disorder	1.00	Excellent	Excellent	Excellent
Major depressive disorder	0.92	Excellent	Excellent	Excellent
Social phobia	0.91	Satisfactory	Excellent	Excellent
Post-traumatic stress disorder	0.90	Satisfactory	Excellent	Excellent
Panic disorder	0.85	Satisfactory	Excellent	Excellent
Psychotic disorder	0.82	Satisfactory	Excellent	Excellent
Substance use disorder	0.81	Satisfactory	Excellent	Excellent
Dysthymic disorder	0.75	Satisfactory	Excellent	Very good
Bipolar I disorder	0.73	Satisfactory	Fair to good	Very good
Specific phobia	0.73	Satisfactory	Fair to good	Very good
Other bipolar (II or NOS)	0.65	Unacceptable	Fair to good	Very good
Generalized anxiety disorder	0.55	Unacceptable	Fair to good	Good

organization of this variability are taken into account. Indeed, usually reliability research starts from the basic assumption that mental distress is expressed via symptoms and signs that univocally refer to underlying disorders. Within this line of reasoning, diagnosticians screen for specific indicators. For example, loss of appetite and frequent crying are usually seen as indicators of major depression. However, it might be that in patients' experience of distress and in the accounts they give about their mental suffering, varying symptoms come to the fore. For example, at one moment an individual might feel sad, while at another concerns about physical health or anxious preoccupation with people's opinions come to the fore. Obviously, symptoms and complaints don't simply appear and disappear on a daily basis, but the weight that is subjectively attributed to specific symptoms, and the narratives along which distress is communicated, might indeed vary quite substantially.

If this is the case, it is not so surprising that in the study of Chmielewski et al. (2015), the evaluations of interviews with a one-week interval, and a second interviewer who creates a different interactional context, yield results that are so dissimilar from the research condition in which a single audiotaped interview is used.

Thus, research into diagnostic reliability has inadvertently opened another field of inquiry: what psychiatric disorders exactly are and how mental health symptoms can be conceptualized. In discussions about diagnosis and assessment it is often argued that reliability is a necessary condition for validity. Indeed, before we can ever conclude that an instrument measures the phenomenon we want it to, we must already be convinced that the instrument yields stable results. Reliability research on the DSM sheds doubt on its scientific credibility, but this should not make us shy away from the issue of validity and from examining how psychopathology is best conceptualized. The next chapter deals with this topic.

Conclusion

An important conclusion that can be drawn from the results presented in the previous section is that the reliability of contemporary DSM-based diagnosis is exaggerated, and not based on evidence. Large-scale studies that propose to demonstrate its superiority in relation to diagnosis, as practiced prior to the publication of the DSM-III, are not only lacking, but in fact the kappa coefficients for inter-rater reliability point to the opposite, suggesting that clinical diagnosis is no more reliable than it was in the 1950s, 1960s, and 1970s. Obviously, some diagnostic categories are now rated more consistently than they were before. For example, whereas in pre-DSM-III times problems were observed in the diagnosis of psychophysiological reactions (see Table 2.2: kappa = 0.38), complex somatic disorders are now diagnosed in much more reliable ways (see Table 2.9: kappa = 0.61). Conversely, other disorders used to be diagnosed more reliably than they are now, which goes against the *fantasy* of substantial progress in the parade of DSM editions. For example, whereas before DSM-III the diagnosis of alcoholism was very reliable (see Table 2.2: kappa = 0.71) the current diagnosis of alcohol use disorder is substantially more ambiguous (see Table 2.9: kappa = 0.40).

According to Jacques Lacan (1949) the stories people tell in order to make sense of their actions have a defensive function. They are selective in nature and serve the function of obfuscating the nonsensical elements, powerlessness, and discord that lie at the basis of our actual experience of the world. More particularly, the ego qua self-reflective agent fulfills this obfuscating role.[16] In my opinion, the now dominant account of psychiatric diagnosis serves a similar role. It tells a heroic story that in pre-DSM-III times diagnosis was unscientific. Yet, thanks to the enlightened neo-Kraepelinians, diagnosis has been safeguarded from bias and is now ready to enter a neurogenetic revolution. Such reasoning not only fortifies a belief in the power of psychiatry, but also obfuscates the very obvious and fundamental problems at the heart of diagnostic decision-making.

In the 1960s and 1970s, empirical studies, including those of Maurice Temerlin and David Rosenhan, cast a shadow on psychiatric diagnosis, arguing that all kinds of subjective factors on the side of the clinician had a radical impact and distorted the decisions made. Critical scholars such as Michel Foucault further added to this point. Foucault pointed out that diagnoses are reifications of a somewhat magical nature, which function, above all, to install disciplinary and controlling power regimes. Indeed, one of the central issues these critics expose concern the uncontrolled impact emanating from the clinician's subjectivity on the conclusions they draw. Since those days, *the fact that clinicians are fallible human beings makes up the Achilles heel of psychiatry*. The neo-Kraepelinian movement and the architects of the DSM obfuscated this problem, suggesting that by following sound procedures and focusing on strictly observable behaviors the subjectivity of the clinician could be filtered out. They acted as if, conditional upon being dipped in the river Styx sufficiently well, Achilles doesn't have a vulnerable heel. Research on diagnostic reliability, by contrast, demonstrates that this approach has failed spectacularly: diagnostic decisions are still just as dependent on individual choices as they ever

---

[16] Lacan indicates that next to playing this obfuscating role the ego is nonetheless crucial to the experience of mental consistency.

were. Obviously, this confronts us with an epistemic problem. On the one hand, the knowledge clinicians construct in their daily practice is marked by idiosyncrasies that cannot be left out of consideration. On the other hand, disorders might not be the kind of stable underlying condition that reifying interpretations bring to the fore.

Apart from flagrantly continuing to ignore this problem, two other options are open. On the one hand, the future of diagnosis could be sought in a further exclusion of subjectivity through more radical strategies of standardization: clinicians are fallible beings, so in order to diminish their subjective impact, protocols and computer-assisted procedures should be introduced. To put it differently: amputate Achilles feet and replace them with prostheses so that he is no longer vulnerable. On the other hand, a solution might be sought at the level of dealing with the idiosyncrasies and flaws in human reasoning. This strategy aims at acknowledging one's points of weakness and helping Achilles deal with them.

In his essay "Why I Do Not Attend Case Conferences," Paul Meehl comments that despite academic training, clinicians tend to be sloppy thinkers: their lines of reasoning are marked by logical fallacies, they use all kinds of self-serving biases, they tend to justify themselves instead of putting their conclusions to the test in their collegial discussions, they underestimate the value of systematic work, and, finally, they systematically neglect the insights of their peers. Meehl observed these problems even before the appearance of the DSM-III, yet in contemporary clinical practice the same problems return. Research on how people reflect on DSM disorder categories demonstrates that similar fallacious lines of reasoning permeate our current age of criteria-based diagnosis (see Tait 2009). Instead of denying these issues or covering them up with protocols, clinicians could be schooled in handling the elements that undermine their credibility. This not only requires education in logical thinking (Croskerry 2003; Kahneman 2011) and the art of rhetoric and debate, but also requires clinicians to reflect on the personal idiosyncrasies they are affected by. In this context, supervision in clinical practice is essential, but not sufficient. What is of key importance here is that before attributing all kinds of characteristics to other people, trainees should explore the dark corners of their own minds. They should become acquainted with the anxieties, desires, and prejudices that determine the decisions they make as well as the actions they take. Indeed, the practice of diagnosis should value more strongly the *craft of clinical reasoning*. This doesn't mean excluding subjective decision-making but recognizing it and subjecting it to reasonable control. Obviously, such an interest in *the craft of clinical reasoning* doesn't lie at the basis of the DSM. Returning to the *Statistical Manual for the Use of Institutions for the Insane*, classificatory diagnostic instruments were above all developed on the basis of administrative concerns. They aimed at *quantifying* mental distress but neglected the way in which clinicians *qualitatively judge* the object/subject they are concerned with. A new era of psychiatric diagnosis should move away from the classificatory approach and emphasize the clinical process between diagnosticians and their patients.

Other References

Angermeyer, M. C., Holzinger, A., Carta, M. G., & Schomerus, G. (2011). Biogenetic explanations and public acceptance of mental illness: Systematic review of population studies. *The British Journal of Psychiatry, 199*, 367–372.

Angst, J. (2002). Historical aspects of the dichotomy between manic-depressive disorders and schizophrenia. *Schizophrenia Research, 57*, 5–13.

Baer, L., & Blais, M. A. (2010). *Handbook of clinical rating scales and assessment in psychiatry and mental health*. New York: Humana Press.

Batstra, L., & Thoutenhoofd, E. D. (2012). The risk that DSM-5 will further inflate the diagnostic bubble. *Current Psychiatry Reviews, 8*, 260–263.

Beck, A. T., Ward, C. H., Mendelson, M., Mock, J. E., & Erbaugh, J. K. (1962). Reliability of psychiatric diagnoses: 2. A study of consistency of clinical judgments and ratings. *American Journal of Psychiatry, 119*, 351–357.

Ben-Zeev, D., Young, M. A., & Corrigan, P. W. (2010). DSM-V and the stigma of mental illness. *Journal of Mental Health, 19*, 318–327.

Bergmann, J. R. (1992). Veiled morality: Notes on discretion in psychiatry. In P. Drew & J. Heritage (Eds.), *Talk at work: Interaction in institutional settings* (pp. 137–162). Cambridge: Cambridge University Press.

Berrios, G. E., & Hauser, R. (1988). The early development of Kraepelin's ideas on classification: A conceptual history. *Psychological Medicine, 18*, 813–821.

Bleuler, E. (1934). *Textbook of psychiatry*. New York: Macmillan.

Carey, B. (2008, December 17). Psychiatrists revise the book of human troubles. *New York Times*.

Chmielewski, M., Bagby, R. M., Clark, L. A., & Watson, D. (2015). Method matters: Understanding diagnostic reliability in DSM-IV and DSM-5. *Journal of Abnormal Psychology, 124*, 764–769.

Clarke, D. E., Narrow, W. E., Regier, D. A., et al. (2013). DSM-5 field trials in the United States and Canada, part I: Study design, sampling strategy, implementation, and analytic approaches. *American Journal of Psychiatry, 170*, 43–58.

Compton, W. M., & Guze, S. B. (1995). The neo-Kraepelinian revolution in psychiatric diagnosis. *European Archives of Psychiatry and Clinical Neuroscience, 245*, 196–201.

Cosgrove, L., & Krimsky, S. (2012). A comparison of DSM-IV and DSM-5 panel members' financial associations with industry: A pernicious problem persists. *Plos Medicine, 9*, e1001190.

Cosgrove, L., Krimsky, S., Vijayaraghavan, M., & Schneider, L. (2006). Financial ties between DSM-IV panel members and the pharmaceutical industry. *Psychotherapy and Psychosomatics, 75*, 154–180.

Cosgrove, L., Krimsky, S., Wheeler, E. E., et al. (2014). Tripartite conflicts of interest and high stakes patent extensions in the DSM-5. *Psychotherapy and Psychosomatics, 83*, 106–113.

Croskerry, P. (2003). The importance of cognitive errors in diagnosis and strategies to minimize them. *Academic Medicine, 78*, 775–780.

Dar-Nimrod, I., & Heine, S. J. (2011). Genetic essentialism: On the deceptive determinism of DNA. *Psychological Bulletin, 137*, 800–818.

Decker, H. (2007). How Kraepelinian was Kraepelin? How Kraepelinian are the neo-Kraepelinians? – from Emil Kraepelin to DSM-III. *History of Psychiatry, 18*, 337–360.

Decker, H. (2013). *The making of DSM-III*. New York: Oxford University Press.

DeFife, J. A., Peart, J., Bradley, B., et al. (2013). Validity of prototype diagnosis for mood and anxiety disorders. *JAMA Psychiatry, 70*, 140–148.

Dehue, T. (2008). *De depressie-epidemie. Over de plicht het lot in eigen hand te nemen [The depression epidemic. On the duty to control your own destiny]*. Amsterdam: Augustus.

Dowrick, C. (2009). *Beyond depression: A new approach to understanding and management*. Oxford: Oxford University Press.

Feighner, J. P., Woodruff, R. A., Winokur, G., Munoz, R., Robins, E., & Guze, S. B. (1972). Diagnostic criteria for use in psychiatric research. *Archives of General Psychiatry, 26*, 57–63.

First, M. B., Spitzer, R. L., Gibbon, M., et al. (1995). The structured clinical interview for DSM-III-R personality disorders (SCID-II). Part II: Multi-site test-retest reliability study. *Journal of Personality Disorders, 9*, 92–104.

First, M. B., Williams, J. B. W., Karg, R. S., & Spitzer, R. L. (2016). *Structured clinical interview for DSM-5 disorders – Clinican version (SCID-5-CV)*. Washington, DC: American Psychiatric Association.

Fleiss, J. L., & Cohen, J. (1973). The equivalence of weighted kappa and the intraclass correlation coefficient as measures of reliability. *Educational and Psychological Measurement, 33*, 613–619.

Fleiss, J. L., Levin, B., & Paik, M. (1981). The measurement of interrater agreement. In J. L. Fleiss, B. Levin, & M. C. Paik (Eds.), *Statistical methods for rates and proportions – Third edition* (pp. 598–626). New York: Wiley.

Foucault, M. (1965). *Madness and civilization: A history of insanity in the age of reason*. New York: Random House.

Foucault, M. (2006 [1973–1974]). *Psychiatric power – Lectures at the Collège de France*. New York: Picador.

Frances, A. (2012, May 8). *Newsflash from APA meeting: DSM-5 has flunked its reliability tests*. Retrieved May 19, 2013, from http://www.huffingtonpost.com/allen-frances/DSM-5-reliability-tests_b_1490857.html.

Frances, A. (2013). *Saving normal – An insider's revolt against out-of-control psychiatric diagnosis, DSM-5, big pharma, and the medicalization of ordinary life*. New York: William Morrow & Harper Collins Publishers.

Freedman, R., Lewis, D. A., Michels, R., et al. (2013). The initial field trials of DSM-5: New blooms and old thorns. *American Journal of Psychiatry, 170*, 1–5.

Gagnon, M. A., & Lexchin, J. (2008). The cost of pushing pills: A new estimate of pharmaceutical promotion expenditures in the United States. *PLoS Med, 5*(1), e1.

Grandin, T. (2013). *The autistic brain – Thinking across the spectrum*. Boston: Houghton, Mifflin Harcourt.

Grob, G. N. (1987). The forging of mental health policy in America: World War II to new frontier. *Journal of the History of Medicine and Allied Sciences, 42*, 410–446.

Grob, G. N. (1991). Origins of DSM-I: A study in appearance and reality. *American Journal of Psychiatry, 148*, 421–431.

Guze, S. B. (1992). *Why psychiatry is a branch of medicine*. New York: Oxford University Press.

Haggerty, G., Zodan, J., Zubair, A., et al. (2016). Reliability and validity of prototype diagnosis for adolescent psychopathology. *The Journal of Nervous and Mental Disease, 204*, 287–290.

Harper, D. (2011). *Online etymological dictionary*. Retrieved September 7, 2011, from http://www.etymonline.com/index.php?search=diagnosis.

Harwood, V. (2010). Mobile asylums: Psychopathologisation as a personal, portable psychiatric prison. *Discourse: Studies in the Cultural Politics of Education, 31*, 437–451.

Haslam, N. (2011). Genetic essentialism, neuroessentialism, and stigma: Commentary on Dar-Nimrod and Heine (2011). *Psychological Bulletin, 137*, 819–824.

Healy, D. (2008). Historical overview: Kraepelin's impact on psychiatry. *European Archives of Psychiatry and Clinical Neuroscience, 248*(Suppl 2), 18–24.

Hiller, W., Dichtl, G., Hecht, H., et al. (1993). An empirical comparison of diagnoses and reliabilities in ICD-10 and DSM-III-R. *European Archives of Psychiatry and Clinical Neuroscience, 242*, 209–217.

Hyman, S. E. (2010). The diagnosis of mental disorders: The problem of reification. *Annual Review of Clinical Psychology, 6*, 155–179.

Kahneman, D. (2011). *Thinking, fast and slow*. New York: Farra, Strauss & Giroux.

Kant, E. (1764/2011). Essay on the maladies of the head. In P. Frierson & P. Cuyer (Eds.), *Emmanuel Kant: Observations on the feeling of the beautiful and sublime and other writings*. Cambridge: Cambridge University Press.

Keller, M. B., Hanks, D. L., & Klein, D. N. (1996). Summary of the DSM-IV mood disorders field trial and issue overview. *The Psychiatric Clinics of North America, 19*, 1–28.

Kirk, S. A., & Hsieh, D. K. (2004). Diagnostic consistency in assessing conduct disorder: An experiment on the effect of social context. *American Journal of Orthopsychiatry, 74*, 43–55.

Kirk, S. A., & Hsieh, D. K. (2009). Do perceptions of dysfunction and normality mediate clinicians judgments of adolescent antisocial behavior? *Social Service Review, 83*, 245–266.

Kirshner, L. (2009). Biopolitics and the transformation of the psychiatric subject. In S. Binkley & J. Capetillo (Eds.), *A Foucault for the 21st century: Governmentality, biopolitics and discipline in the new millennium* (pp. 92–104). Newcastle upon Tyne: Cambridge Scholars Publishing.

Klerman, G. L. (1978). The evolution of a scientific nosology. In J. C. Shershow (Ed.), *Schizophrenia: Science and practice* (pp. 99–121). New York/London: Guilford.

Kraemer, H. C., Periyakoil, V. S., & Noda, A. (2002). Tutorial in biostatistics: Kappa coefficients in medical research. *Statistical Medicine, 21*, 2109–2129.

Kraepelin, E. (1907). *Clinical psychiatry* (p. 1981). Delmar: Scholars' facsimiles and reprints.

Kraepelin, E. (1921). *Manic-depressive insanity and paranoia*. Edinburgh: Livingstone.

Kutchins, H., & Kirk, S. A. (1997). *Making us crazy: DSM – The psychiatric bible and the creation of mental disorders*. New York: Free Press.

Kvaale, E. P., & Haslam, N. (2016). Motivational orientations and psychiatric stigma: Social motives influence how causal explanations relate to stigmatizing attitudes. *Personality and Individual Differences, 89*, 111–116.

Kvaale, E. P., Haslam, N., & Gottdiener, W. H. (2013). The 'side effects' of medicalization: A meta-analytic review of how biogenetic explanations affect stigma. *Clinical Psychology Review, 33*, 782–794.

Lacan, J. (1988 [1953–1954]). *The seminar of Jacques Lacan, book I: Freud's papers on technique*. New York/London: W.W. Norton.

Lacan, J. (1988 [1954–1955]). *The seminar of Jacques Lacan, book II, the ego in Freud's theory and in the technique of psychoanalysis*. Cambridge: Cambridge University Press.

Lacan, J. (2006 [1949]). The mirror stage as formative of the function of the I. In J. Lacan & J. A. Miller (Eds.), *Écrits* (pp. 75–81). New York/London: W. W. Norton.

Laing, R. D. (1960). *The divided self: An existential study in sanity and madness*. Harmondsworth: Penguin.

Landis, J. R., & Koch, G. G. (1977). The measurement of observer agreement for categorical data. *Biometrics, 33*, 159–174.

Lane, C. (2008). *Shyness: How normal behavior became sickness*. Yale: Yale University Press.

Maj, M. (2012). Validity and clinical utility of the current operational characterization of major depression. *International Review of Psychiatry, 24*, 530–537.

McNally, R. J. (2011). *What is mental illness?* Cambridge/London: Belknap Harvard.

Meehl, P. E. (1973). Why I do not attend case conferences. In *Psychodiagnosis: Selected papers* (pp. 225–302). Minneapolis: University of Minnesota Press.

Menninger, K. A. (1959). The psychiatric diagnosis. *Bulletin of the Menninger Clinic, 23*, 226–243.

Menninger, K., Ellenberger, H., Pruyser, P., & Mayman, M. (1958). The unitary concept of mental illness. *Bulletin of the Menninger Clinic, 22*, 4–12.

Moskowitz, A., & Heim, G. (2011). Eugen Bleuler's Dementia praecox or the group of Schizophrenias (1911): A centenary appreciation and reconsideration. *Schizophrenia Bulletin, 37*, 471–479.

Moynihan, R., Heath, I., & Henry, D. (2002). Selling sickness: The pharmaceutical industry and disease mongering. Commentary: Medicalisation of risk factors. *BMJ, 324*, 886–891.

Mukolo, A., Heflinger, C. A., & Wallston, K. A. (2010). The stigma of childhood mental disorders: A conceptual framework. *Journal of the American Academy of Child and Adolescent Psychiatry, 49*, 92–198.

Nietsche, F. (1887). *The gay science*. New York: Vintage Books.

Nieweg, E. H. (2005). On reification and natural kinds in psychiatry. *Tijdschrift voor Psychiatrie, 47*, 687–696.

Parens, E., & Johnston, J. (2011). Troubled children: Diagnosing, treating and attending to context: A hastings center special report. *Hastings Center Report, 41*(2), 1–32.

Peerenboom, E. (2002). Transparent science. *EMBO Reports, 3*(1), 9–11.

Philips, C. B. (2006). Medicine goes to school: Teachers as sickness brokers for ADHD. *Plos Medicine, 3*, e182.

Pickard, H. (2009). Mental illness is indeed a myth. In L. Bortolotti & M. Broome (Eds.), *Psychiatry as cognitive science: Philosophical perspectives* (pp. 83–101). London: Open University Press.

Pigeaud, J. (2001). *Aux portes de la psychiatrie. Pinel, l'ancien et le moderne*. Paris: Aubier.

Pinel, P. (1806). *A treatise on insanity*. Sheffield: Todd.

Pottick, K. J., Kirk, S. A., Hsieh, D. K., & Tian, X. (2007). Judging mental disorder in youths: Effects of client, clinician and contextual factors. *Journal of Consulting and Clinical Psychology, 75*, 1–8.

Rafalovich, A. (2004). *Framing ADHD children: A critical examination of the history, discourse, and everyday experience of attention deficit/hyperactivity disorder*. Lanham: Lexington Books.

Regier, D. A., Narrow, W. E., Clarke, D. E., et al. (2013). DSM-5 field trials in the United States and Canada, part II: Test-retest reliability of selected categorical diagnoses. *American Journal of Psychiatry, 170*, 59–70.

Robins, E., & Guze, S. (1970). Establishment of diagnostic validity in psychiatric illness: Its application to schizophrenia. *American Journal of Psychiatry, 126*, 983–987.

Rose, N. (1996). *Inventing our selves – Psychology, power and personhood*. Cambridge: Cambridge University Press.

Rose, N. (1999). *Governing the soul – The shaping of the private self – Second edition*. London/New York: Free Association Books.

Rosen, G. M., & Lilienfeld, S. O. (2008). Posttraumatic stress disorder: An empirical evaluation of core assumptions. *Clinical Psychology Review, 28*, 837–868.

Rosenhan, D. (1973). Being sane in insane places. *Science, 179*, 250–258.

Rosenhan, D. (1975). The contextual nature of psychiatric diagnosis. *Journal of Abnormal Psychology, 84*, 462–474.

Scheff, T. (1966). *Being mentally ill – A sociological theory*. Chicago: Aldine.
Schomerus, G., Schwahn, C., Holzinger, A., et al. (2012). Evolution of public attitudes about mental illness: A systematic review and meta-analysis. *Acta Psychiatrica Scandinavica, 125*, 440–452.
Skre, I., Onstad, S., Torgensen, S., & Kringlen, E. (1991). High interrater reliability for the structured clinical interview for DSM-III-R Axis I (SCID-I). *Acta Psychiatrica Scandinavica, 84*, 167–173.
Solomon, A. (2012). *Far from the tree – Parents, children and the search for identity*. London: Vintage books.
Spitzer, R. L. (1975). On pseudoscience in science, logic in remission and psychiatric diagnosis: A critique of Rosenhan's 'on being sane in insane places'. *Journal of Abnormal Psychology, 84*, 442–452.
Spitzer, R. L., & Fleiss, J. L. (1974). A re-analysis of the reliability of psychiatric diagnosis. *British Journal of Psychiatry, 125*, 341–347.
Spitzer, R. L., Endicot, J., & Robins, E. (1978). Research diagnostic criteria – Rationale and reliability. *Archives of General Psychiatry, 35*, 773–782.
Spitzer, R. L., Forman, J. B. W., & Nee, J. (1979). DSM-III field trials: I. Initial interrater diagnostic reliability. *American Journal of Psychiatry, 136*, 815–817.
Spitzer, R. L., Williams, J. B., Gibbon, M., & First, M. B. (1984). *Structured clinical interview for DSM-III axis I disorders*. New York: New York State Psychiatric Institute.
Strand, M. (2011). Where do classifications come from? The DSM-III, the transformation of American psychiatry, and the problem of origins in the sociology of knowledge. *Theory and Society, 40*, 273–313.
Szasz, T. S. (1961). *The myth of mental illness – Foundations of the theory of personal conduct*. New York: Harper & Row.
Tait, G. (2009). The logic of ADHD: A brief review of fallacious reasoning. *Studies in Philosophy and Education, 28*, 239–254.
Temerlin, M. K. (1968). Suggestion effects in psychiatric diagnosis. *Journal of Nervous and Mental Disease, 147*, 349–353.
Temerlin, M. K. (1970). Diagnostic bias in community mental health. *Community Mental Health Journal, 6*, 110–117.
The Psychologist. (2011). Society's critical response to DSM-5. Retrieved Oktober 17, 2013, from http://www.thepsychologist.org.uk/blog/blogpost.cfm?threadid=2102&catid=48.
Timimi, S., & Leo, J. (2009). *Rethinking ADHD*. London/New York: Palgrave MacMillan.

Trajkovic, G., Starcevic, V., Latas, M., et al. (2011). Reliability of the Hamilton rating scale for depression: A meta-analysis over a period of 49 years. *Psychiatry Research, 189*, 1–9.

Van Os, J. (2016). "Schizophrenia" does not exist. *The British Medical Journal, 352*, i375.

Van Os, J., Kenis, G., & Rutten, B. P. (2010). The environment and schizophrenia. *Nature, 268*, 203–212.

Van Os, J., Rutten, B. P., Myin-Germeys, I., et al. (2014). Identifying gene-environment interactions in schizophrenia: Contemporary challenges for integrated, large-scale investigations. *Schizophrenia Bulletin, 40*, 729–736.

Vanheule, S., Desmet, M., Meganck, R., et al. (2014). Reliability in psychiatric diagnosis with the DSM: Old wine in new barrels. *Psychotherapy and Psychosomatics, 83*, 313–314.

Viera, A. J., & Garrett, J. M. (2005). Understanding interobserver agreement: The kappa statistic. *Family Medicine, 37*, 360–363.

Weber, M. M., & Engstrom, E. J. (1997). Kraepelin's "diagnostic cards". The confluence of clinical research and preconceived categories. *History of Psychiatry, 8*, 375–385.

Welner, A., Liss, J. L., & Robins, E. (1974). Systematic approach for making a psychiatric diagnosis. *Archives of General Psychiatry, 31*, 193–196.

Westen, D. (2012). Protoype diagnosis of psychiatric syndromes. *World Psychiatry, 11*, 16–21.

Westen, D., DeFife, J. A., Bradley, B., & Hilsenroth, M. J. (2010). Prototype personality diagnosis in clinical practice: A viable alternative for DSM-5 and ICD-11. *Professional Psychology: Research and Practice, 41*, 482–487.

Williams, J. B. W., & Kobak, K. A. (2008). Development and reliability of a structured interview guide for the montgomery depression rating scale (SIGMA). *British Journal of Psychiatry, 192*, 52–58.

Williams, J. B. W., Gibbon, M., First, M. B., et al. (1992). The structured clinical interview for DSM-III-R (SCID) – II. Multisite test-retest reliability. *Archives of General Psychiatry, 49*, 630–636.

Woodruff, R., Goodwin, D., & Guze, S. (1974). *Psychiatric diagnosis*. New York: Oxford University Press.

Zanarini, M. C., Skodol, A. E., Bender, D., et al. (2000). The collaborative longitudinal personality disorders study: Reliability of Axis I and II diagnoses. *Journal of Personality Disorders, 14*, 291–299.

Ziółkowska, J. (2012). The objectifying discourse of doctors' questions. Qualitative analysis of psychiatric interviews. *Social Theory & Health, 10*, 292–307.

3

Symptom and Context: The Issue of Validity in Diagnosis

Toward a Functional Account of Psychopathology

The question as to how to diagnose a mental condition is as old as the question of how to treat it, and throughout history all kinds of procedures, rituals, and technologies have been explored. Diagnosis is well rooted in knowledge about psychopathology, but at the same time it is often seen as a clinical art, one which requires well-trained clinicians with a good eye for subtle signs of illness. Going against the idea of diagnosis as simply a factual and mechanistic undertaking that is merely concerned with observing and assessing signs of mental disturbance, this chapter addresses the assumptions underlying common ideas about symptoms and disorders. Particular attention is paid to the question of how *context* plays a role in diagnosis. A main argument I make is that in the DSM, the context of the individual (i.e., the personal life history, social circumstances, cultural background) is thought to play only a *minor moderating role* in relation to symptom formation and expression. Indeed, the manual mainly follows a sign-based logic, which coheres with the assumption that biological irregularities are to be found at the basis of mental distress. I argue that by doing so the DSM cultivates a rather naïve essentialistic view on mental disorders, which not only fuels reification but also obfuscates the fact that the DSM rests on pragmatic grounds. At the same time, I make a plea for a *self-reflexive and contextualizing* account of psychopathology. Such a viewpoint doesn't neglect problem-specific or disorder-specific regularities, but assumes that typical configurations never unequivocally apply to single cases, thus necessitating a casuistic approach to diagnosis.

Practically speaking, diagnosis in the DSM is pretty straightforward: using standardized sets of inclusion and exclusion criteria for each disorder, the diagnostician reviews the patient's complaints and decides which diagnosis is indicated. Indeed, pivotal to DSM-based diagnosis are the brief checklists that are formulated for each disorder. These include key symptoms, specifications on the minimal duration of complaints, and indications of other conditions that might provoke similar symptoms. In total, the DSM-5 discerns 347 mental disorders (spanning 677 pages) grouped into 20 broad categories, such as "depressive disorders," "neurocognitive disorders," and "schizophrenia spectrum and other psychotic disorders."

Next to these checklists, the DSM also contains brief descriptions of each disorder. These descriptions outline the diagnostic features of a given disorder (i.e., its development and course, prevalence, differential diagnosis relative to other conditions, and comorbidity), which provide a slightly broader framework for interpreting the information contained in the checklists. Nonetheless, the DSM focuses on grouping mental symptoms in syndromal disorder clusters, paying less attention to characteristic illness dynamics and typical psychopathological processes.

How the DSM Takes into Account Context

Notwithstanding its rather static focus on the disorder features that make up clinical pictures, the attentive reader of the DSM-5 might notice the commentary on the use of the manual, wherein one paragraph (DSM-5, p. 19) is devoted to the relation between diagnosis (based on standard criteria) and the use of contextual information. Here it states that while the use of diagnostic criteria is necessary to "assure a more reliable assessment" (a dubious claim we examined in Chap. 2), they are not sufficient to make a diagnosis. In order to properly grasp "the relative severity and valence of individual criteria and their contribution to a diagnosis," "clinical judgment" is needed. Details concerning what this clinical judgment precisely is, in the context of the DSM, and how severity and valence should be taken into account are unfortunately not given. However, one point the manual puts forth is that diagnosis should be linked to *clinical case formulation*: "The case formulation for any given patient must involve a careful clinical history and concise summary of the social, psychological, and biological factors that have contributed to developing a given mental disorder." By taking such information into account, the clinician should develop a balanced idea of the problems or symptoms the individual is affected by, which should ultimately lead to a balanced clinical intervention: "The ultimate goal of a clinical case formulation is to use the available contextual and diagnostic information in developing a comprehensive treatment plan that is informed by the individual's cultural and social context."

Next to this commentary on the use of clinical case formulation and subsequent treatment planning, the DSM-5 (pp. 749–759) contains a ten-page section on cultural issues. This section discusses how cultural contexts may influence illness experience and symptom expression and provides an assessment instrument called the *Cultural Formulation Interview* (CFI). This interview is designed to detect the cultural identity of the interviewee; typical cultural conceptualizations of distress that might shape his or her distress; psychosocial stressors and cultural features of vulnerability and resilience; and cultural specificities of the relationship between the individual and the clinician.

At first sight, promoting the use of contextual information and encouraging cultural case formulation in the process of clinical decision-making might be applauded: finally, DSM diagnosis takes into account the human being as well the context beyond the symptoms. This is a timely development. After all, several key psychiatrists note that in clinical practice the DSM is often used in reductive ways. For example, in an editorial in the *American Journal of Psychiatry* the editor in chief at that time,

Nancy Andreasen (2001, p. 674), notes the following: "Unfortunately, our fast-moving cyberworld threatens to separate us from our roots and to tempt us to forget our origins. Many of us are besieged by injunctions to interview and diagnose patients as quickly as possible, and sometimes even to eliminate our 'old-fashioned' and 'inefficient' narrative records that summarize present illness and past history, replacing them with checklists of diagnostic criteria and symptom ratings." All too often diagnosis tends to be reduced to pigeonholing complaints, whereby time-consuming activities, such as careful clinical and cultural case formulation, do not fit the agenda of the psychiatrist. This remark reminds us of an older study from the pre-DSM-III era (Sandifer et al. 1970), which observed that long before the checklist approach came into vogue, ordinary diagnostic decision-making tended to be overhasty. In an experimental setting, the researchers examined how psychiatrists make inferences from videotaped diagnostic interviews. The conclusion was sobering: contrary to the image of the carefully listening analyst, psychiatrists used very little information from the tape before drawing conclusions and, moreover, seemed to have already made up their minds within minutes after the beginning of the interview (Verhaeghe 2002). Unfortunately, times haven't really changed: diagnoses still tend be made "as quickly as possible" (Andreasen 2001, p. 674). Against the background of this tendency to rapidly come to conclusions, the recent appeal to use contextual and diagnostic information in clinical case formulation seems progressive.

However, the plea to make use of contextual information in DSM diagnosis is not new. A similar, yet brief, call to embed diagnostic classification in a broader exploration of illness dynamics can already be found in the DSM-III (pp. 11–12). In the Introduction, the DSM task force, or more specifically its chairman Robert Spitzer (Decker 2013), noted: "Making a DSM-III diagnosis represents an initial step in a comprehensive evaluation leading to the formulation of a treatment plan" (DSM-III, p. 11). Yet, as Andreasen (2001) suggests, diagnosis frequently remains restricted to the initial step, concluding with labels for individuals in terms of categories of disorder. This is not surprising: brief introductory notes on the combined use of diagnosis and case formulation simply cannot sufficiently guide diagnostic practice. They pay lip service to the idea that the person beyond the diagnosis is important, but actually lay the foundation for completely misrecognizing all that is person-specific, just as they neglect the relation between, on the one hand, symptoms, and on the other hand, social situations and (sub-)cultural backgrounds. If diagnosis is to be contextualized, precise ideas on the relationship between symptom and context must be developed.

Adding half-hearted sections on the issue of case formulation doesn't solve the problem. The reflections on cultural case formulation and the *Cultural Formulation Interview* from the DSM-5 illustrate this. Obviously, the interview is meant as a tool for diagnosing non-Western individuals. Yet, a commentary as to why and how a North American instrument like the DSM is applicable in different cultures cannot be found in the manual. For example, the DSM-5 (p. 20) contains a definition of a mental disorder, but it doesn't question the pertinence of such a definition in different cultures, where issues of individual mental health might have a different status than it has had in the past decades in the USA. Even a statement on how dominant discourses in the West affect illness experience in the Western world is lacking; it is as if shifting viewpoints of mental distress, changing socio-economical practices, and broader epistemological positions do not affect symptom expression and experience. What is also missing in the DSM is a theoretical position on how cultural case formulation should actually be used in different cultures. Anthropological research reveals that Western illness concepts tend to disrupt non-Western cultural practices in their management of mental distress (e.g., Watters 2010). Diagnostic manuals like the DSM, which "expert" Western practitioners flagrantly apply in different cultures, provide individuals with diagnoses that do not match their local customs. Bluntly or subtly, local illness accounts are treated as inferior to Western ideas (Good 1994). Diagnostic practices tend to enact the classic colonial attitude, in which "bad" situations are solely observed, evaluated, and treated from a Western moral and epistemological framework. As such approaches often have a bewildering effect in local contexts (e.g., Trudgen 2000), it would be appropriate that the DSM not only pays attention to cultural case formulation, but also provides reflective sections on the cultural and social position of the DSM using psy-professional, and on the value of the manual across cultural and social settings. Specifically, a section dedicated to the ways in which knowledge and power tend to function in the psy-disciplines[1] might also make clinicians more thoughtful about the psychosocial function of diagnoses.

Let's return to the DSM-5 Introduction, and take a closer look at how this so-called case formulation is said to be related to diagnosis. According to the manual, in making a diagnosis the "clinical history" as well as a "summary of the social, psychological, and biological factors" that may have contributed to the disorder should be considered, such that "the relative severity and valence" of the checklist criteria can be taken into account (DSM-5, p. 19). A question that this statement raises, however, is precisely how to conceive the relation between symptom and contextual factors. I propose that *in the DSM context is thought to play a minor moderating role in relation to symptom formation and expression.* This perspective can be contrasted with the viewpoint that symptom and context make up an indivisible systemic whole. However, first we will take a closer look at the classificatory process underlying the DSM.

The Paradox of Polythetic Descriptive Diagnosis

Characteristically, the DSM provides checklists for diagnosing mental disorders in a *descriptive* and *polythetic* way. Each disorder is defined in terms of inclusion and exclusion criteria, based on which a professional can decide from which disorder a person is suffering. This decision-making process is based on a list of *descriptive* features of each disorder; with an inventory of symptoms the diagnostician explores whether a given individual meets a sufficient number of the inclusion criteria as well as certain specifications that would exclude the diagnosis of a particular disorder. In other words, the specific complaints with which the individual presents are translated in psychiatric jargon, and situated relative to a taxonomic classification of possible disorders, and the clinician must evaluate whether the presenting symptoms are signs of one or more disorders. For example, for major depressive disorder the DSM-5 lists nine relevant

---

[1] Good discussions of power and discipline in contemporary psy-professions can be found in the works of Ian Parker (2010) and Nikolas Rose (1996, 1999).

clinical characteristics. Major depressive disorder can be diagnosed if at least five criteria are present, with the proviso that at least one of the symptoms includes either depressed mood or loss of interest or pleasure. For each DSM-5 disorder, the same template of inclusion and exclusion criteria is used. Some disorders exclude one another; for example, a diagnosis of major depressive disorder excludes schizoaffective disorder, while other disorders might be combined, pointing to comorbidity, like major depressive disorder with comorbid generalized anxiety disorder.

Since the checklist-based approach was adopted, the DSM follows a *polythetic* system: it sketches broad profiles for most disorders, which implies that people with the same disorder might actually have completely different symptom profiles. Within the logic of polythetic diagnosis it is assumed that such variation is not cause for concern due to the obvious "family resemblance" between different symptom profiles: all symptoms more or less point to the same underlying category (Berrios 1999, 2012, p. 102). The strength of polythetic diagnosis is that it covers variability: patients with different symptomatic profiles can be classified into one category. Such grouping is unproblematic as long as all patients within the same category still share key features. The weakness of polythetic diagnosis, by contrast, is that such diversity is subsumed under a general nominator and as a result the more specific features that characterize individual cases fade into an abyss of irrelevance. Moreover, binary polythetic diagnosis only establishes whether symptoms are present or not. This obfuscates the extent to which the given list of descriptors actually grasps the nature of the individual's complaint. The DSM-5 partly solved this problem by adding dimensional severity scales for clusters of symptoms for some disorders. For example, this is the case for autism spectrum disorder and alcohol use disorder, but not for major depressive disorder or schizophrenia. Most importantly, a detailed network analysis in which it was examined to which extent symptoms contribute to broader disorder categories shows that individual DSM symptoms differ substantially in their association with the diagnostic category they should belong to (Boschloo et al. 2015). Each symptom has a unique valence and value, and therefore is not interchangeable with other symptoms. This finding contradicts the idea that diagnoses can validly be made by just counting the number of symptoms.

Just as its two predecessors, the DSM-5 continues to use the polythetic classification principle in an as rigorous way as ever. As such, it is more than likely that two individuals with the same diagnosis have only a few, and occasionally no, traits in common. For instance, in the case of schizophrenia it might be that one individual obtains the diagnosis due to having hallucinations and disorganized speech, and another because of delusions and negative symptoms (i.e., diminished emotional expression or avolition) (see DSM-5, p. 99). In major depressive disorder, it is possible that one individual is diagnosed due to the presence of depressed mood, weight loss, insomnia, psychomotor agitation, and fatigue, while another is given the same diagnosis due to the presence of diminished interest in most daily activities, recurrent thoughts of death, diminished ability to concentrate, feelings of worthlessness, and hypersomnia (see: DSM-5, pp. 160–161): one disorder, two entirely different symptom profiles. Indeed, for the majority of DSM diagnoses patients with entirely different symptom profiles might be classified in the same disorder category. Such rigorous application of the polythetic classification principle might function as a source of unreliability. Moreover, Lilienfeld and Marino (1999, p. 400) suggest that notwithstanding the use of diagnostic checklists in the DSM, disorder categories function as "Roschian concepts." This means that based on the disorder criteria, diagnosticians try to agree on "an ideal mental prototype that embodies the central features of the category." Yet as the polythetic principle is applied it is quite likely that different diagnosticians consider different features as central to a disorder. This might bring them to building a different diagnosis for the same individual.[2]

Given the fact that since the DSM-III the American Psychiatric Association defines all mental disorders in purely descriptive terms, such an extreme polythetic approach is rather paradoxical. In the DSM-III it was argued that for most mental disorders the etiology was actually unknown, which gave rise to the well-known descriptive approach: "the definitions of the disorders generally consist of description of the clinical features of the disorders. […] This descriptive approach is also used

---

[2] Thusly so, Westen's (2012) plea for a return to explicit prototype-based diagnosis as an alternative should be taken seriously.

in the division of the mental disorders into diagnostic classes. All of the disorders without known etiology or pathophysiological process are grouped together on the basis of shared clinical features" (DSM-III, p. 7). Following this logic, one would expect that disorder descriptions build on a common set of mandatory symptoms and that variation is only possible in terms of additional features. Indeed, if a disorder is nothing more than the sum of specific symptoms, irrespective of its underlying processes and etiology, one would expect that in two individuals with the same diagnosis, common symptoms prevail. However, this is not the case in the DSM. The examples of schizophrenia and major depressive disorder show that two individuals with the same diagnosis might not actually share any symptoms at all. This brings us to the paradox: if disorders are defined based on the presence of a specific number of descriptive features only, how is it possible for two individuals to have the same disorder if they have none of the clinical features in common? This paradox has important consequences in terms of the validity of a DSM diagnosis. Diagnostic categories can only be considered as valid if the constituent cases are sufficiently alike and mutually coherent, referring to a similar underlying clinical reality. Extreme polythetic classification weakens diagnostic coherency, thus undermining diagnostic validity.

Sign-Based Diagnosis

One characteristic of the DSM approach to diagnosis is that the professional first attends to an individual's complaints and subsequently translates them into standard psychiatric language. This is illustrated in the *Structured Clinical Interview for DSM Disorders* (SCID). In the SCID interview, the diagnostician doesn't permit the interviewee to express his problems in the idiom he would normally make use of, but reviews all DSM criteria to ascertain whether they apply to what the patient presents. The SCID interview, like the DSM, is carefully designed to avoid the (messy) idiosyncratic representations and ideas that characterize an individual's experience of psychopathology. For example, in the context of making a diagnosis of premenstrual dysphoric disorder it is asked whether in the week before onset of the menses a woman experiences "marked irritability or anger or increased interpersonal conflicts," and whether these "symptoms" improve within few days after onset (DSM-5, p. 172). In making a DSM diagnosis one examines *whether* such a criterion applies to an individual.

In doing so, it is assumed that laypersons and trained professionals can sufficiently agree on how they define "irritability," "anger," and "interpersonal conflict." Likewise it is taken for granted that they use corresponding standards for assessing what can be defined as "marked" irritability, and that they use comparable thresholds in determining whether the psychological state one experiences as "marked" is actually abnormal or pathological. What is not explored is the question as to *how* and under what circumstances this would be the case. Variation in terms of contextual psychosocial factors and in how an individual lives through her complaint is left completely out of consideration. Moreover, no attention is paid to the manner in which the individual interprets or weaves meaning around her experience.

Following the semiotic theorist and novelist Umberto Eco (1976), such an approach bears witness to a neopositivist approach to psychical distress. In such an approach it is assumed that specific symptoms are relatively stable and unambiguous indicators of an underlying condition. Considered from the perspective of medical semiotics, the DSM assumes that symptoms are *signifiers* that can be linked to a fixed *referent*. In semiotic theory, the *signifier* refers to the physical carrier of information (Eco 1976). Examples of signifiers are multiple, ranging from written letters and spoken sound to icons on doors or red lights on the corner of a street. Likewise, behavioral, verbal, and bodily expressions can be understood as signifiers of distress. The referent, in its turn, is the physical object, event, action, or illness to which a signifier refers (Eco 1976). For example, the material object I press my fingers on as I type is the referent of the signifier "keyboard." In the DSM, the disorders that the system discerns are the referents to which the inclusion and exclusion criteria qua signifier refer. Each of the 347 referents in the system is accompanied by unique but overlapping sets of signifiers that should give rise to unambiguous diagnoses.

More specifically, the DSM seems to start from the belief that symptoms are so-called *indexical signifiers*, or *signs*. This means that, following the logic of the DSM, the relationship between signifier and referent is not only fixed, but also causal in nature: the disorder as referent causes the manifestation of the symptom qua signifier. This is what I conclude from the suggestion that the criterion sets "*point* to an underlying disorder" (DSM-5, p. 19, my italics). Within the DSM a potential patient is seen as the sender of signifiers of illness, which the diagnostician qua receiver must decode. For this decoding process to be successful it is crucial that the receiver possess the code whereby the signifiers can be linked to the correct referent. In psychiatric diagnostics, as performed within the DSM, the handbook with its list of disorders and their criteria makes up such code (Vanheule 2012).

As indicated, the note on clinical case formulation in the DSM-5 suggests that a "summary of the social, psychological, and biological factors" might be relevant in diagnosis since it allows the practitioner to grasp "the relative severity and valence" of the checklist criteria (DSM-5, p. 19). In semiotic terms, this seems to imply that such factors are significant in terms of how they alter or moderate signal strength. The DSM-5 doesn't actually specify this, but if we follow this line of reasoning one might, for example, expect that personality characteristics influence the way in which symptoms are expressed. A particularly extrovert person might communicate complaints differently than an extremely introverted person, and be more dramatic and expressive. The person's overall style thus moderates the way the symptom is expressed, but doesn't alter the nature of the symptom itself. A similar line of reasoning could be applied to how innate temperamental characteristics or social class influence symptom expression: such factors modify the form of the symptom but don't affect its inherent qualities. Within this line of reasoning, symptoms resemble natural objects like vegetables: depending on the circumstances in which lettuce is grown (in a garden or in a greenhouse; near the equator or near the polar circle) its shape, color, and taste might differ, but it is still just lettuce. Similarly, context variables might shape the form of symptoms, but the moderating effect these variables have is inconsequential for the nature of the symptom itself. Indeed, social, psychological, and biological factors might add noise to the disorder signs the sender is transmitting, but these factors do not change the indexical relation between the symptom qua signifier and the disorder qua referent.

Beyond Sign-Based Diagnosis: Symptoms as Personal Constructions

Interestingly, semiotic theory discerns a third component in its study of the human use of signs: the *signified*. The signified is the concept or idea that humans connect to their use of signifiers. Signifieds are created as humans try to make sense of the world, attribute meanings, and build mental representations. Whereas the signifier qua material carrier of information and the referent qua object, event, or action are transindividual, this doesn't seem to be the case for the signified. Signifieds are created by sense-making individuals, and their content depends on the precise way in which a person interprets the signifiers he uses and perceives. In the DSM the signified connected to the signifiers of distress does not receive attention. It is assumed that, above all, the sense connected to symptoms is a common sense: laypersons and trained professionals are believed to have the same signified in mind when they discuss specific symptoms.

The question is whether such focus on the sign-like quality of mental symptoms and the neglect of the dimension of the signified in psychiatric diagnosis is justified. If this is not the case, the study of how individuals use signifiers in making sense of their own suffering should be more central to the study of psychopathology.

An important characteristic of the DSM's descriptive classificatory diagnosis is that it merely deals with the human being qua observable object. What it disregards is that people also always have a *reflexive relation* to their own actions and symptoms. The phenomenologist[3] Josef Parnas (2012, p. 120) articulates this as follows: "the human being is *both* an empirical object and a transcendental subject, that is a condition of possibility for its own study." An individual living through a difficult period and experiencing a plethora of symptoms is not simply the sum of these problems. He is also always the relation to his own suffering and to the context within which this suffering came to the fore. This reflexive relationship implies that, invariably, people *interpret* the elements of the

---

[3] Sometimes the DSM's focus on description is characterized as "phenomenological" (e.g., Decker 2013). This is confusing since the phenomenological approach to psychopathology, as illustrated by the quote of Parnas, largely exceeds the DSM-like focus on description.

distress that they experience. Interpretation determines the sense or nonsense people attribute to their experience of distress, and guides them in qualifying their distress as a problem or not.

For example, research in the general population indicates that many people report anomalous psychological experiences: In a British sample of 1000 individuals Pechey and Halligan (2012) observed that 48 % of the sample reported occasional or frequent anomalous or paranormal experiences. These experiences were significantly associated with the presence of beliefs of a delusional nature, which were also quite common: 39 % of the participants reported strong belief in ideas of a delusional nature, and 25 % reported strong beliefs in bizarre ideas of a delusional nature (Pechey and Halligan 2011). However, such beliefs and experiences are often not reported to cause distress and thus deemed unrelated to psychopathology (Evrard 2013). Similarly, in various international surveys, Beavan et al. (2011) observed that approximately 13.2 % of people from the general population occasionally hear voices. From a purely descriptive point of view, it might be concluded from these studies that large numbers of individuals have plainly psychotic or attenuated psychotic symptoms. Yet, without taking into account the effect of the voice on the voice-hearer, or of the belief on the believer, such conclusions are unjustifiable. After all, most people from the general population who hear voices are not distressed (Kelleher et al. 2010; Van Os 2010). Neglecting the subjective aspect of the individual's experiences is ill starred as it leads to a one-sided appraisal of mental health problems (Stoyanov et al. 2012). Taking into account the reflexive relation people have to their own symptoms implies that *the subject* and[4] *subjective* experience are crucial to what

---

[4] It is important to note that within various philosophical traditions the concepts of subjectivity and subject obtain different interpretations. For example, in phenomenological approaches, subjectivity is identified with conscious experience as the fundamental ground of our understanding of both the world and ourselves. This dimension of conscious experience is considered to be accessible through self-reflection, based on which a person can construct a narrative about what he lives through. In this view subjectivity is knowable and, eventually, amenable to a normative evaluation (is this person's self-experience adequate or not?). From a Lacanian psychoanalytic point of view, by contrast, the subject qua product of self-reflexivity is not a discernible entity but a self-relating "emptity." Self-related thoughts and speech connote who we are and what we live through, but never denote the subject. Within this view the notion of the subject refers to the multitude of signifiers, based on which self-experience is constituted and across which self-experience is fundamentally scattered; hence the idea that the subject is "divided." Lacan does not think of the subject as a psychological

a symptom is for a person. There is a real danger that if the subject and subjective experience are not explicitly taken into account, especially for individuals that are not particularly communicative or are easily intimidated by psy-professionals, only a partial appraisal of distress is made.

If *symptom experience* was more central to diagnosis the mere presence of descriptive characteristics would be less of an issue. As Jim Van Os (2010, p. 308) suggests, such an alternative approach to diagnosis "in part becomes understanding the onset of *need for care*." The study of human psychological functioning teaches us that that there is quite some variety in how people behave. Yet variation comes in degrees, making some behaviors and mental phenomena more uncommon than others. Certain ways of behaving and relating that resemble the kind of symptoms often reported by patients might seem peculiar, but should not give rise to diagnosis if they don't provoke distress. Mental states should only be of clinical concern if they are not (or no longer) manageable for a person. This is reminiscent of Freud's (1913) suggestion that symptoms come in varieties. In his view, most people, if not all, carry symptoms, albeit some suffer more than others. Throughout time, symptoms can obtain a different status. At some moments a symptom might be part of a person's habitual mode of functioning, working as a livable compromise between incompatibilities the person is living with, such as conflicting desires or incongruities between desires and inhibitions. At other moments, the balance can lean toward the other side: compromises then obtain a pathological quality and start to produce more distress than tranquility (Verhaeghe 2002). Consequently, the important question a diagnostician needs to ask concerns the factors that made the balance keel to the other side, prompting a request for help. By disregarding symptom experience DSM-based diagnosis neglects such questions.

Against this criticism, it could be argued that in the end the DSM-5 does take into account the reflexive relation people have to their symptoms. After all, it asks diagnosticians to pay attention to symptom

---

or teleological instance that makes use of signifiers, but as the connotative effect of using signifiers. The subject doesn't produce speech; speech produces the subject. Thus considered, self-reflexivity does not imply self-transparency. On the contrary, from a Lacanian point of view self-reflexivity is marked by an impossibility, which makes up the unconscious. Nevertheless, what both philosophical traditions have in common is the explicit valorization of subjectivity.

severity and valence: aren't these attempts to grasp precisely how a person experiences distress? Perhaps they are. But obviously people's reflexive relationships to their symptoms is only of secondary importance in the DSM. In terms of the comment made by Parnas (2012), the DSM above all qualifies mental disorders as empirical objects to which all transcendental subjectivity is subordinated. This bears witness to a *naturalistic* attitude. Indeed, in the DSM the self-reflexive relation is not considered to be *constitutive* of mental symptoms; it is a factor that may moderate their expression, but by no means organizes them.

Ivana Marková and German Berrios (2009) formulate interesting challenges for such a naturalistic approach (see also Berrios and Marková 2002, 2006).[5] In their view, the structures or realities underlying mental symptoms and subjective complaints are basically unstable. Material objects such as vegetables or tables have a relatively constant configuration. They always consist of the same constituents that have a constant functional relation to one another. The appearance of such objects might be altered by contextual variables, like climatological circumstances for vegetables or designers' ideas for tables, but contextual influences don't change the fundamental qualities of the objects. Such is not the case for mental symptoms. The structure of a self-reported mental state, such as "depressed mood," is fundamentally fuzzy because it depends on the individual judgment of the person experiencing that state. What one person qualifies as a depressed mood is not the same as what another individual refers to with the same word. Indeed, mental symptoms are not simply signs of underlying disorders, but above all *personal constructs*: "They are *constructs* in the sense that subjects create sense or construct a meaning out of an inchoate pre-conceptual and preverbal experience. They are *personal* in that, although social and cultural influences will help their articulation, the experiences themselves are unique to the individual and inaccessible to anyone else" (Marková and Berrios 2009, p. 344). The authors also argue that observed symptoms and behaviors psychiatrists typically take into account when judging an individual's state of mind cannot be considered as entities with a stable structure: "This time the

---

[5] Interesting psychometric challenges for the DSM approach to mental symptoms can be found in the work of Denny Borsboom and colleagues (e.g., Borsboom and Cramer 2013).

constructs involved relate to the judgments made by clinicians and we have seen how these will depend on manifold factors (e.g. experience, personal biases and mood) which, being neither fixed nor consistent, will serve to destabilize the structure itself" (Marková and Berrios 2009, p. 346).

Following this viewpoint it could be argued that by a priori separating symptoms from the lived context of an individual, and not asking clinicians to take into account the personal meaning-making processes, the DSM makes a big leap. The DSM assumes that symptoms and aspects of personal experience do not make up a systemic whole and can easily be separated. In line with Marková and Berrios I believe this is deeply problematic as it neglects the personal-constructional side of a symptom. In terms of the DSM, lived experience is only a minor moderator: it affects the magnitude or quantity of the symptom, but leaves its quality unaddressed. The question as to how a symptom functions in the context of a person's life, and how exactly or why precisely he is affected in the way that he is, is left out of consideration. Therefore, the DSM decontextualizes mental suffering because it disconnects the symptom from the personal-construction process in which mental suffering is embedded.

In their *Cambridge Model of Symptom Formation*, Berrios and Marková (2006) don't merely treat context as a moderating variable, but as a constructive force in the creation of mental symptoms. In their view, symptoms are made up of both brain signals, which cohere with broader neurophysiological processes, and semantic configuration processes. Central to their conceptual model is the idea that symptoms rest on brain signals that undergo mental elaboration, which are eventually conveyed in clinically observable modes of expression, as we see in self-reported complaints (e.g., "I feel sad," "I hear voices") or clinically observable behaviors (e.g., catatonic stupor, agitation). The model discerns four pathways, sequentially termed (a), (b), (c), and (d) along which brain signals are expressed.

Pathway (a) describes the trajectory along which self-reported symptoms are constituted. It assumes that brain signals "resulting, for example, from a malfunctioning pathway or site or indeed nonpathological firing" first penetrate awareness and create a vague pre-linguistic, preconceptual state of consciousness called the "primordial soup" (Berrios and Marková

2006, p. 31). Although they don't discuss this explicitly, it is quite likely that in order to give rise to symptomatic expression, the primordial soup should provoke feelings of unease and malaise. The model says that in a next step the person interprets his state of mind and configures it "in terms of personal, familiar, social, and cultural formats" (Berrios and Marková 2006, p. 31). The configuration process implies a procedure of transformation along which the primordial soup is encoded in a multi-layered world of ideas, images, and meanings, which can be communicated. Obviously, this transformation process is complex and influenced by the person's habitual ways of speaking about experiences and the body, in which personal, familial, social, as well as (sub-)cultural factors can be discerned. In their discussion of the elements that influence the configuration of the primordial soup, Berrios and Marková (2006, p. 32) state:

> "Various factors are likely to be important, for example, the social and cultural background of the individual, past experiences of like events, general and personal knowledge and attitudes, contexts in which it takes place, familial styles of response, and so on. In addition, it is likely that the interpretation and articulation of the resultant symptom will be further influenced by individual language capacity, imagination, decision as to whether to express, and, importantly, the effect of interacting with an interlocutor (often the clinician)."

The net result is that, although based on a brain signal, a symptom can hardly be seen as the direct expression of a neurobiological reality.

Pathway (b) in the Cambridge Model of Symptom Formation describes the way in which clinically observed symptoms that don't give rise to subjective complaints are constituted. Characteristic of these symptoms is that specific brain signals don't generate a primordial soup entering awareness, but are immediately expressed in behavioral manifestations, which the diagnostician might interpret as signs of an underlying condition. This time the component of interpretation is not on the side of the patient, but on the side of clinician, who must evaluate whether or not the observable traits in the patient's functioning signal a disorder.

Pathway (c) is used to describe vague unnamed symptoms. Characteristic of this trajectory is that the brain signal gives rise to the primordial soup, but not to the broader configuration process described in pathway (a). In this case, the patient is aware of mental or somatic distress, but fails to make sense of these subjective experiences, that is, name and classify them in terms of relevant culturally and socially sanctioned modes of expression. The clinician in his turn might learn about such distress via vague complaints in which the experience of unease stands to the fore.

Pathway (d) in its turn describes a path leading to symptoms that are not rooted in a disturbed neurobiological signal. This pathway makes clear that some symptoms are secondary in nature and are provoked by primary symptoms that are indeed an expression of brain signals: "some symptoms may be viewed as secondary constructions. For example, anxiety may develop secondary to a frightening hallucination" (Berrios and Marková 2006, p. 33). The idea here is that primary symptoms may trigger an individual's configuration processes, thus provoking secondary symptoms. The model indicates that especially disorganized psychological functioning and the presence of aberrant images in the mind might prompt the creation of such secondary symptoms.

What is interesting about the Cambridge Model of Symptom Formation is that, contrary to how the DSM approaches symptoms, it underscores the formative and configuring role of context on symptoms, ranging from personal life history, familial influences, and social factors to cultural determinants. The model does not deny the role of neurobiological factors, but considers them as fundamentally intertwined with context variables.

However, on a different note, it could be argued that the conceptual model of Berrios and Marková could be criticized for being too linear. For example, at the level of pathway (a) they assume that brain signals create a primordial soup in consciousness, which is then configured in terms of relevant context variables, thus giving rise to symptoms. What they don't seem to model is how important feedback loops might be added between the different pathway components. These would shed a different light on causality. In pathways (a), (b), and (c) of the Cambridge Model of Symptom Formation, brain signals make up the first step in symptom formation, which suggests that in the end most distress is essentially neurobiological. By adding feedback loops to the model, causality could be thought of as more circular in nature. For example, from a sociological point of view it might be argued that perceived inequality in a given society is an important cause of mental disorders (Verhaeghe 2014; Wilkinson and Pickett 2009). In terms of the model, this implies that a feedback loop should be drawn between configuration processes and brain signals: perceiving oneself as disadvantaged in relation to others might provoke brain signals that give rise to distress. Another reason why a feedback loop could be added in between configuration processes and brain signals has to do with important individual differences in *how* individuals make sense of distress. From a psychoanalytic point of view, it can be argued that in dealing with their distress, some people have a strong tendency to negate and repress, while others are inclined to face and analyze their problems and act upon them. These different styles of managing distress likely have a different impact on the distress as well as on the brain signal that initially gave rise to distress: negation and repression have a worsening effect, while facing and analyzing distress are alleviating. Indeed, more broadly, it could be argued that the effect of psychotherapy, which has a profound impact on brain functioning (e.g., Buchheim et al. 2013; Karlsson 2011), might be thought of as a feedback loop going from configuration to brain signal and distress.

Moreover, the Cambridge Model of Symptom Formation assumes that symptoms are always *provoked* by biological signals: construction processes transform the brain signal that gives rise to distress but in the end, the biological component is the "prime mover." This is also true for pathway (d), which describes ancillary symptoms that rest on primary, that is, biologically caused, symptoms. Against or complementary to such a naturalizing view it might be argued that symptoms can also have a psychological or psychosocial cause, which then provokes biological irregularities. For example, experiences such as falling in love, losing a best friend, or being disappointed as a parent can provoke psychological processes that are primal in relation to biological disturbances. In these cases the trigger is non-biological, while its effect will obviously be mirrored in the body. As he makes a plea for recognizing *psychical causality*, Lacan refers to *identification* (Lacan 1947) and signification processes in relation to life events (Lacan 1959) as potential triggers for setting illness processes in motion. Although starting from a completely different perspective, behaviorists, in their attention to learning processes driven by external stimuli, also point to modes of causality that are not primarily biological (Moore 2001). By adding psychical causality to the pathways of the Cambridge Model of Symptom Formation this model changes. What is thus created is a *Systemic Model of Symptom Formation*, which assumes that the causal factor could be situated at each level that the model discerns.

However, my main objection toward the Cambridge Model of Symptom Formation is that it only maps the dimensions that determine symptom formation, thus neglecting the processes by which a symptom is constructed. For example, the model acknowledges that individuals configure the primordial soup they experience in terms of personal, familiar, social, and cultural formats, suggesting the symptom obtains "an onionlike structure in which the primordial soup is wrapped in multiple layers of meaning" (Berrios and Marková 2006, p. 31). Yet, how are these "multiple layers of meaning" constituted? And how do "forms" and "styles of talking" produce their constitutive effect on both the primordial soup and the symptom? It is through the act of speaking, thinking, and fantasizing about who one is and what one lives through. In this context, the verbal and pragmatic embedment of mental symptoms in speech acts should be stressed, which is not the case in the Cambridge Model of Symptom Formation.

In de Saussure's (1916) structural linguistics, a distinction is made between three constitutive dimensions: speech, language, and individual speaking. In his view, speech (*langage* in French) concerns the rule-abiding game humans play when communicating via linguistic signs. Language is transindividual, and concerns our ability to communicate and reflect in an orderly way by means of lexical and grammatical conventions and rules. Language (*langue* in French), by contrast, is a specific tongue, or a specific system of linguistic signs and grammatical rules an individual uses to express something. For example, English or French are languages. Indeed, whereas speech refers to the abstraction of human language use, language concerns the specific idiom one makes an appeal to. Individuals assimilate language, such that in a next step they can use it to write, talk, and reflect. Speaking (*parole* in French), in its turn, concerns an individual's specific speech acts, which are expressed in a certain way, with specific stylistic and interactional qualities. Whereas language is a collectively shared social product, which no one masters completely and entirely, speaking is an individual's product, which can be observed in the practical ways language is used. Language is virtual: it can be mapped in dictionaries and other documents, but even when it is not formally documented it exists. Speaking, by contrast, is actually graspable in specific linguistic expressions. Note that in de Saussure's work, speaking has a rather broad meaning, referring to all kinds of specific utterances, verbal or written.

What is interesting about the distinction between speech, language, and speaking is that it draws our attention to *structural* and *pragmatic* aspects of how individuals use linguistic signs. Speech and language make up structural frameworks individual speakers rely upon. Specific speech acts concretize and actualize the general systems of speech and language, using these as a treasure trove from which elements are selected at the moment an individual speaks. In his work, de Saussure describes speech as a general ability humans have, and language as a social construction and a specifically shaped tongue that a community of speakers relies upon. In his view, language is strongly synonymous with the different languages (e.g., French, English) we discern, meaning that the collective level he concentrates upon is the language community in its very general form. Yet language communities might be thought of as far more local: ICT specialists in Mumbai use English in different ways than inhabitants from a small Scottish village; college graduates use language differently compared people with lower schooling; subcultures employ different slang; and families have their own habitual narrative styles. Indeed, next to cultural, social, and familial contexts, each individual has their own style, which is determined by life events, learning processes, and memories. Indeed, ultimately each individual makes up a language community that is composed of different internal voices, and these styles can be mapped. When language communities are compared, we map general patterns, pointing to structural differences and similarities between the units being compared.

In the Cambridge Model of Symptom Formation the aspect of configuration seems to refer only to such structural and stylistic characteristics.

Consequently, the model strongly presents the symptom as a *product* of multiple contextual influences (personal, familial, social, cultural), which at the level of language make up different language communities. Yet, perhaps the *speech act* itself is the most important context in which the symptom needs to be situated. Symptoms cannot be seen as fixed things. Indeed, in their later work Marková and Berrios (2009) stress that symptoms are personal constructs. If this is the case, the way symptoms are constructed in the process of speaking should be more central in how mental symptoms are modeled. When an individual complains of depression it doesn't suffice to get hold of the social, cultural, familial, and individual meanings she attributes to such a state. We principally gain knowledge of her depressive mood because she talks about it. Thus it is in the speech act that the symptom is articulated and defined. However, the exact form of the articulation will contain variability, such as subtle thematic variations, temporal shifts in style, or vaguely contradictory claims. Apart from this, the speech act also expresses non-verbal characteristics, including intonation, hesitation, and scansion. In the speech act some narrative lines about the symptom might be particularly well elaborated, while others are poor and ambiguous. Moreover, speaking is not only the activity through which the symptom is expressed, it is also the process through which it might be challenged, questioned, and redefined. Indeed, just as neurophysiological and configuring processes modulate the characteristics of the mental symptom, speaking also shapes its characteristics.

Therefore, as an alternative to the Cambridge Model, I present the *Triangular Model of Symptom Formation* (see Fig. 3.1). This model proposes that the symptom is best conceptualized as an outcome of three systemically connected processes: the act of speaking, within which meaning arises and non-verbal markers are expressed; neurophysiological processes, which might give rise to an explicit occurrence of unease and malaise, or not; and contextual influences that provide a general framework within which experience is configured. At the level of these contextual factors we situate the structural impact of language on mental functioning. Within this model, the symptom is a multidimensional product with certain speech-act specific qualities, biological characteristics, and contextual configuration features covering characteristics that are specific of an individual, family, social context, and (sub-)culture.

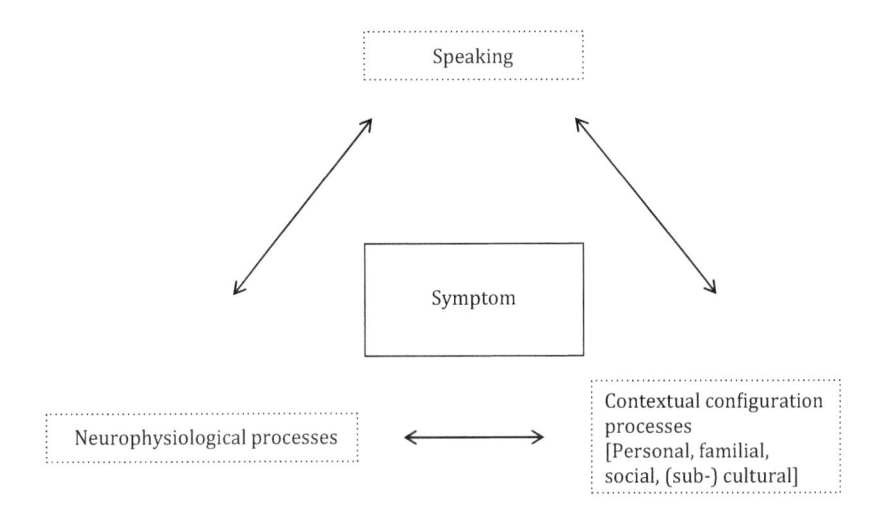

3 Symptom and Context: The Issue of Validity in Diagnosis

Fig. 3.1 Triangular model of symptom formation

Intermezzo: Lacan's Position

A minimal conclusion we can draw from the previous section is that separating symptoms from subjective experience and the meaning-making processes that get shaped via speech acts is unjustifiable. Psychiatric diagnosis should start from a clinical theory in which the *signified* that is constructed around and via mental symptoms is taken into account, assuming that such signifieds get created within the chain of signifiers speech acts produce. In the work of Lacan (1957, 1959) such theory can be found.

One characteristic of Lacan's work is that he thinks of mental symptoms in terms of speech and language: on the one hand, speech and language enable the human being to name what he lives through in speech acts, and thus to signify himself as a subject. Indeed, the principal way in which clinicians gain knowledge of patients' symptoms is through speaking: people speak about their problems, and by listening as well as asking questions diagnosticians learn about symptoms and about the effect these symptoms have on people's self-experience. Yet, on the other hand, Lacan also stresses that all attempts at signifying mental suffering fundamentally fall short: some aspects, which he qualifies as *Real*, cannot be named and insist in symptoms. Indeed, the human use of language is marked by a gap, by elements of nonsense and stupefaction that interfere with our effort to make sense of what we live through.

Throughout his work, Lacan frequently refers to three dimensions or registers that make up mental life and also compose mental symptoms: the *Symbolic*, the *Imaginary*, and the *Real*. Human beings function in the register of the Symbolic to the extent that they make use of signifiers. These are not only the material building blocks of language, but also the foundation of mental life as such (Lacan 1957): all mental representation rests on the distinctions we make by means of signifiers. Characteristic of the Symbolic is that it makes up the register via which (sub-) cultural, social, and familial habits and laws get articulated. The Imaginary, in its turn, is made up of the ideas or signifieds language use creates. By means of language, we build images on how the world is and on who we are. Given the fact that meaning implies the creation of a mental image, which people tend to focus on, Lacan considers it as Imaginary (Vanheule 2011). In developing these ideas on the signifier and the signified Lacan builds on the work of Ferdinand de Saussure (1916). Yet, whereas de Saussure believed that people make use of language in order to communicate signifieds, Lacan stressed that meaning principally arises contextually through speaking. Meaning is not an a priori given but created by linking signifiers in so-called signifying chains that make up speech acts and lines of thought.

As we apply Lacan's distinction between these three registers to mental symptoms, they can be conceptualized as having a symbolic, imaginary, and a real component. Symptoms are symbolic to the extent that they are determined by language-based configuration processes, and are constituted via speech acts. The imaginary component concerns the signifieds and ideas that get associated to symptoms. These have both a personal side—for example, for a specific individual, voice hearing is related to the day her mother left for another partner and she began to hear voices—and a collective component, implying that shared meanings are associated with specific symptoms—for example, in terms of hearing voices: shared opinions on madness or paranormal activity might come to the fore in how an individual makes sense of such a symptom. Yet above all, symptoms often have a shocking effect. They destabilize the ideas and feelings a person holds about himself and the world, introducing an element of unpredictability and strangeness in the heart of self-experience. In Lacanian terminology this is the *real* component of the symptom, which, for example, is expressed in the stupefaction and anger an individual might express while thinking about or relating personal problems. Note that this Lacanian account of the symptom specifically aims at characterizing the experience of the symptom, meaning that causal factors, like biological, psychological, or socio-cultural causes, are not included in it.

As a consequence, in order to study the subjective impact of the symptom, diagnosis should above all start from the specific way in which the symptom is embedded in the act of speaking. On the one hand the process of diagnosis should study the way in which a person talks about his problems and complaints, and expresses distress. On the other hand it should get hold of the issues and meanings the symptom is associated with. Thus considered, diagnosis has a double focus: it aims at studying both the *particularities* and *singularities*[6] in speech.

Diagnosis is focused on *particularities* insofar as it aims at detecting the *type of psychopathology* a person suffers from. In Lacan's approach, types of psychopathology are studied in terms of underlying structures in speech, called *clinical structures* (Nobus 2000; Parker 2010; Verhaeghe 2002). The names Lacan gives to these structures cohere with traditional psychiatric discourse, for example, discerning neurosis, psychosis, and perversion. Yet, rather than thinking of clinical structures as *underlying* disorders or illness realities to which symptoms refer, Lacan studies psychopathology in terms of how the Real, the Symbolic, and the Imaginary are organized in a person's functioning, and how this eventually coheres with mental suffering. In terms of the Cambridge Model of Symptom Formation this means that Lacan is particularly concerned with diverse patterns at the level of configuration processes. Indeed, what is interesting about Lacan's theory is that it helps us discern different ways of dealing with the Real, the Symbolic, and the Imaginary. For example, in

---

[6] The terms *particularities* and *singularities* are often used synonymously. I suggest distinguishing them: "particular" refers to characteristics that hold true for subgroups; "singular" refers to characteristics and events that cannot be generalized.

Lacan's view there is no such thing as a psychotic symptom. A symptom is only thought to be structured in a psychotic way if by speaking about his symptom an individual bears witness to a particular subjective position. Only by taking into account the specific ways in which a person uses signifiers can this position be detected. One such element that is characteristic of the psychotic structure is the experience of perplexity concerning thoughts, observations, or feelings that are qualified as arising out of the blue. Coming from an unimaginable beyond, these create breaches in the continuity of mental life, which baffles the individual (Vanheule 2011). Lacan doesn't connect the question of clinical structure to patterns at the level of biological parameters, but perhaps both lines of reasoning might be combined.[7]

Diagnosis is focused on *singularities* insofar as it takes into account the non-generalizable events, incidents, and memories that mark a person's mental life. Indeed, just as it is unjustified to simply pigeonhole mental symptoms in terms of DSM disorder categories, diagnosis should not simply consist of detecting clinical structures. What a diagnosis should grasp and describe is *how*, through his unique trajectory in life, a person constructs his mental suffering and tries to deal with it. Thus, the signifying process itself must be studied carefully. Since signifiers only make sense in relation to one another in signifying chains, this viewpoint implies that symptoms cannot be studied as snapshots taken out of context. Therefore, the diagnostician should not only attend to the signifiers and signifieds used in speech about symptoms and complaints, but always contextualize them in the narrative of the life history, relationships, existential questions, and the social and cultural circumstances the person lives in. However, it is also at the level of singularity that we

---

[7] Lacanian psychoanalysis does not reject the idea that psychopathology is governed by laws that can be described in scientific terms, but maintains that the reflexive relation an individual has to his own condition cannot be reduced to these laws. This theoretical position does not give rise to an idealist theory of the mind in which non-material mental forces are presumed to be active, but to a so-called *decentered materialism*. Crucial to this Lacanian materialism is the divided subject's relation to the Real (De Vos 2014). In this context, Lacan made a relevant distinction between nature and physics. Nature is that which determines us in how we act and through our self-reflexive attitude we can relate to it. Physics, like all other sciences, is a discourse based on which we study and intervene upon the world. Science constitutes just one way of relating to nature. It transforms our way of relating to nature, but never eliminates what is Real to a subject.

need to situate the register of the Real. Invariably, all meaning-generating signification or configuration processes end up with a deadlock, with nonsensical elements that nonetheless insist at the level of how a person experiences himself and the world. Taking into account the way a person relates to the Real is crucial to a Lacanian-based diagnosis.

What is interesting about this viewpoint is that particularities don't preclude singularities. Ideally both are taken into account in diagnostic discussions with respect to specific cases and symptoms. However, often naturalizing approaches that focus on rigid disorder categories are juxtaposed with personalistic approaches that focus on individualities. By focusing only on disorders and neglecting case-specific characteristics and events, the DSM bears witness to such one-sidedness.

The Search for Biomedical Referents

As indicated above in our discussion of the Cambridge Model of Symptom Formation, the DSM qualifies mental symptoms as signs that point to underlying disorders. Whereas in the DSM-I (1952) and II (1968) no epistemological statements concerning the precise nature of mental disorders can be found, its use of concepts like "neurosis" or "psychological reaction" was highly criticized in the 1970s. Biomedically inspired psychiatrists believed that these labels bore witness of underlying psychological presumptions and, since the DSM-III (1980), succeeded in having them replaced (Decker 2013). In the introduction to the DSM-III, the authors state that "the approach taken in DSM-III is atheoretical with regard to etiology or pathophysiological process" (DSM-III 1980, p. 7). Most interpretations of this phrase focus on the idea that the DSM is neutral in terms of differences between therapeutic schools of thought, like psychoanalysis or cognitive therapy. However, if read to the letter it is a most remarkable phrase. If the statement had been: "atheoretical with regard to etiology *and* pathophysiological process," it would stress theoretical neutrality at both levels. Yet the statement says: "atheoretical with regard to etiology *or* pathophysiological process." In other words, the statement seems to equate etiology and pathophysiology and thus implies that pathophysiological processes, first and foremost, make up mental disorders. What it also says is that at the level of specific neuropsychiatric models and theories, the DSM-III assumes no firm position: no claims are made concerning specific neurobiological disturbances associated to disorders. Such a prioritization of biomedical reasoning is not surprising. After all, most task force members of the DSM-III leaned toward a biomedical approach to psychiatry (Decker 2013).

However, in order to "sell" the DSM to the field of psychiatry, strong epistemological claims on the nature of mental disorders were avoided in the DSM-III, as well as in later editions of the manual. With the advent of the DSM-5 this changed somewhat. The DSM-5 continues to hold on to descriptive criteria; however, disorders are presumed to be biomedical realities more than ever before. While this change is obvious in its preparatory documents, it is subtler in the manual itself. For example, with reference to the motivation to change the DSM-IV-TR, the DSM-5 (p. 5) only mentions cognitive neuroscience, brain imaging, epidemiology, and genetics as relevant background disciplines. Indeed, in line with the basic tenets the so-called neo-Kraepelinian movement formulated in the 1970s (see Chap. 2), basic tenets of biological psychiatric thinking (see Berrios and Marková 2002) guided the development of the DSM-5, like the idea that mental disorders are disorders of the brain caused by biological factors, or the idea that only biologically focused quantitative studies provide relevant scientific insight into the nature of mental disorders.

The process of developing the DSM-5 started in 1999. Key figures involved often indicated that they would drop the descriptive approach and gradually switch to a diagnostic system that was based on a causal understanding of disorders. For example, in 2011 the then president of the American Psychiatric Association, Carol A. Bernstein, wrote: "diagnoses in the DSM-III, DSM-III-R, and DSM-IV are best understood as useful placeholders, based on careful description, but not on deeper understanding" (Bernstein 2011). Guiding the revisions was the attitude that the new handbook should be more strongly informed by scientific innovation—an aim no one can object to—and that the "deeper understanding" that decades of psychiatric research provided would lead to a more objective delineation of the disorder categories. However, the only research addressed during discussions of the new scientific basis for the DSM-5 is, unfortunately, biomedical.

What is iconic in this respect is the edited book *A Research Agenda for DSM-V*. This book intended to be programmatic for all actual revisions: "Those of us who have worked for several decades to improve the reliability[8] of our diagnostic criteria are now searching for new approaches to an understanding of etiological and pathophysiological mechanisms—an understanding that can improve the validity of our diagnoses and the consequent power of our preventive and treatment interventions" (Kupfer et al. 2002, p. xv). The editors, which include DSM-5 chair David Kupfer and vice-chair Darrel Regier, aimed to devise "a research and analytic agenda that would facilitate the integration of findings from research and experience in animal studies, genetics, neuroscience, epidemiology, clinical research, and cross-cultural clinical services[9]—all of which would lead to the eventual development of an etiologically based, scientifically sound classification system." Indeed, key to the DSM-5 revisions was the intention that groundbreaking biomedical findings with respect to etiology and pathophysiology would finally inform diagnostic decision-making. While the DSM-III and the DSM-IV were still merely based on convention, the DSM-5 task force foresaw a near future in which diagnosis would at last be truly valid. In making decisions about inclusion and exclusion criteria they aimed "to carve nature at its joints" (Regier et al. 2009, p. 648). This ambitious claim, which uses a metaphor from Plato's Phaedrus, makes clear that in its classification the DSM-5 assumes that mental disorders are natural kinds, meaning irreducible entities that are rooted in natural laws (Bird and Tobin 2010; Keim Campbell et al. 2011). Thus, the laws thought to be operative are purely *biomedical* and far removed from *psychotherapeutic* or *social psychiatric* assumptions about the processes that make up psychopathology (Bracken et al. 2012; Kirshner 2009; Vanheule 2011).

Indeed, in different publications key figures in the development of the DSM-5 voiced the idea that mental disorders should be thought of as neurobiological entities. According to Stein et al. (2010, p. 1760) the term "mental disorder" is actually misleading and could be replaced by "psy-

---

[8] In Chap. 2 I discuss the fact that this hard work to improve the reliability of psychiatric classification was not particularly successful.

[9] Obviously, these reflections gave rise to the appendix on cultural formulation in the DSM-5.

chiatric disorder" "insofar as it emphasizes that these conditions are not purely 'mental' and that the line between 'psychiatric disorder' and 'other medical disorders' is not distinct." In a collaborative article on the future of psychiatry, the DSM-5 task force chair David Kupfer and colleagues even go a step further and use the term "complex *brain* disorder" instead of "mental disorder" (Reynolds et al. 2009, my italics). In their view, psychiatry is above all a "clinical neuroscience," with the help of which "a deeper understanding of causal pathways to major neuropsychiatric illness is evolving, thus rendering artificial the boundary between psychiatry and neurology" (Reynolds et al. 2009, p. 2), which indeed points to biological psychiatric assumptions (Berrios and Marková 2002). More critically, such a line of reasoning could be seen as illustrative of genetic essentialism and neuroessentialism (Dar-Nimrod and Heine 2011).

However, as the publication date of the DSM-5 approached the tone changed somewhat. In a 2011 commentary in the *American Journal of Psychiatry* the chairs noted the following: "we anticipated that these emerging diagnostic and treatment advances would impact the diagnosis and classification of mental disorders faster than what has actually occurred" (Kupfer and Regier 2011, p. 672). The message they then gave was that biological evidence helped in distinguishing disorders, grouping them into spectra, but did not make up the criteria sets: "While not central to the criteria themselves, this information is nonetheless useful and informative for helping DSM provide a more precise picture of the clinical realities of psychiatric diagnosis" (Kupfer and Regier 2011, p. 672). However, neither in the DSM-5 itself nor in related publications did the DSM task force make clear *which* neurobiological evidence was actually used in making decisions about disorder criteria. Without such detailed information on *how* decades of psychiatric research has informed conclusions about diagnostic categories, the claim that advances in research helped provide a "more precise picture of the clinical realities" is rhetorical. Above all, such lines of reasoning bear witness to what Berrios and Marková (2002) call *the technology alibi*, a rhetorical strategy used since the early nineteenth century in order to support further belief in biomedical illness assumptions:

> "As far as we know, the first person to use the technology alibi was Georget (1820) to explain the failure of biological psychiatry to find any sustainable

and replicable connections between brain and madness. Then, as now, it was only a 'matter of months' before the pathology and genetics of dementia praecox were sorted out; then, as now, the expectation was kept alive by the release of premature data; and then, as now, there was never the scientific honesty of publishing a denial saying that what had been claimed earlier was nonsense" (Berrios and Marková 2002, p. 5).

Despite all rhetoric of grounding the DSM-5 on neurobiological concepts, the manual strongly resembles the previous versions of the handbook and does not read like a rupture with the past: the DSM-5 and the DSM-IV-TR (2000) largely contain the same disorder categories and diagnostic criteria for specific disorders remain mainly the same.[10] This most probably indicates that in the end, empirical research has not been as conclusive as first speculated. After all, the diagnostic categories of the DSM-5 still only contain lists of characteristic symptoms and complaints, which Bernstein (2011) mockingly qualified as "useful placeholders." In other words, despite decades of biologically inspired rhetoric on scientific innovation in psychiatry, not a single "hard" indicator could be included.

Interestingly, other new ideas that had also been launched with reference to "science" were not granted, like the project to assemble existing disorders into larger clusters and spectra. Whereas at first it was indicated that such grouping was "suggested by the scientific evidence" (Bernstein 2011), in the end it was not retained in the handbook. Scientific (or other) arguments as to why the envisioned change was not retained were not communicated.

The net result is that the diagnostic criteria in the DSM-5 are as descriptive as ever before. Nonetheless, the authors of the DSM-5 make the following claim about these criteria: "they are *intended* to summarize characteristic syndromes of signs and symptoms that point to an underlying disorder with a characteristic developmental history, biological and

---

[10] In a 19-page document entitled *Highlights of Changes from DSM-IV-TR to DSM-5* (http://www.dsm5.org/documents/changes%20from%20dsm-iv-tr%20to%20dsm-5.pdf) all changes are reviewed. Nevertheless, several authors, like Allen Frances (2013), correctly suggest that for several disorders inclusion and exclusion criteria were subtly relaxed, thus predicting waves of inflating diagnosis. For example, whereas DSM-IV-TR indicates that a diagnosis of ADHD can be made only if symptoms are present before the age of seven, the DSM-5 indicates that the diagnosis can be made if symptoms are present before the age of 12. This "small" criterion change actually implies that the population eligible for the diagnosis actually doubled.

environmental risk factors, neuropsychological and physiological correlates, and typical clinical course" (DSM-5, p. 19, my italics). Without validity studies actually proving that the polythetic symptom profiles from the DSM correspond to underlying disorders, the above claim is, indeed, no more than an *intention*. An intention is something one aims or hopes for, not something that can be taken for granted. Indeed, straightforward references to validity studies that would substantiate disorder categories are lacking in the DSM-5 and related publications.[11] This means that validity is as much a problem in the DSM-5 as it was in the previous two editions of the handbook.

Why then all the buzz about the scientific basis of the DSM-5 (e.g., Kupfer et al. 2002)? I conclude that, above all, the DSM-5 officials' frequent references to the *idea* of scientific evidence aimed to polish up the credibility of the DSM. The message they seemingly want to sell is that DSM diagnosis should be *thought of* as rooted in sound research, although this is far from clear. Most probably the objective to find a specific and coherent neurobiological structure underlying specific disorders is far too ambitious, except perhaps for neurocognitive disorders (Frances 2013; Kagan 2012; McNally 2011; Van Os 2016).

Toward an Era of Biopsychopathology?

Meanwhile, the US National Institute of Mental Health (NIMH) has created a new project that aims to fill this gap: the Research Domain Criteria (RDoC) project. The aim of this project is to develop a classification of psychopathology or "biopsychopathology" (Kozak and Cuthbert 2016, p. 288) that is based on behavioral indicators, symptoms and neurobiological measures: "RDoC are intended to ultimately provide a framework for classification based on empirical data from genetics and neuroscience" (Insel et al. 2010, p. 749). The idea is that results from biomedical research only have a limited impact on clinical practice because they don't

---

[11] In the process of researching this book I contacted the DSM-5 task force chair and vice-chair, David Kupfer and Darrel Regier, asking both of them whether the scientific studies on the basis of which decisions were made about disorder criteria could be provided. Neither of them responded.

fit in very well with the diagnostic categories of the DSM. The RDoC project, by contrast, aims to create "a framework for research on pathophysiology, especially for genomics and neuroscience, which ultimately will inform future classification schemes" (Insel et al. 2010, p. 748). The project does not immediately focus on disorder categories, but on psychological processes that might be disturbed in case of mental disorder: "narrower psychological constructs such as cognition, emotion, learning, memory, motivation, and perception might be more susceptible to biological analysis than depression, mania, and schizophrenia" (Kozak and Cuthbert 2016, p. 287). Indeed, instead of illness entities, dysfunction at "lower order" psychological processes now makes up the explanandum: "the RDoC approach seeks biological elaboration of intermediate psychological constructs, to yield biopsychological explanations of clinical problems" (Kozak and Cuthbert 2016, p. 288). Most characteristic of the RDoC project is its "biopsychological" focus: by linking research pertaining to psychological processes involved in clinical psychiatric syndromes to insights from pathophysiology, the project aims at creating a framework that will eventually guide clinical practice. Characteristically, RDoC aims at paving the way for an explicitly dimensional perspective on psychopathology: "'biopsychopathology,' eventually might be conceptualized as extremes on psychobiological dimensions that are linked to narrowly determined (in the sense of homogeneity of mechanism) clinical problems" (Kozak and Cuthbert 2016, p. 288).

Currently, the RDoC initiative only provides a framework for research: it delineates key domains of scientific investigation, defining specific areas that researchers should explore, preferably by studying relations between psychological and biological processes and variables: "one of RDoC's operating conventions is to focus on dysfunction in one or more behavioral and brain systems and to relate this to clinical phenomena […] the framework is conceived to facilitate study of circumscribed clinical problems rather than to cluster them into syndromes with larger groups of heterogeneous clinical symptoms" (Kozak and Cuthbert 2016, pp. 294–295). Presently, this framework is still under development, and implications for diagnosis and intervention are unclear. In the meantime it cannot be used for guiding psychiatric diagnosis and treatment. Yet, the hope is that in the end the project will enable the formulation of a nosological classification system that is predicated on a neuroscientific basis and with this outcome the DSM will be further adapted: "we believe this initiative will be very informative for subsequent versions: DSM 5.1, DSM 5.2, and beyond" (Kupfer and Regier 2011, p. 673). Obviously, the timeframe within which such a neuroscientific diagnostic system will be developed is large: "NIMH views RDoC as the beginning of a transformative effort that needs to succeed over the next decade and beyond to implement neuroscience-based psychiatric classification" (Insel et al. 2010, p. 750). Yet, given the fact that such a system is not yet available, the NIMH supports the use of the DSM-5 in clinical contexts (Insel and Lieberman 2013), which is paradoxical, given their profound skepticism toward the validity of the DSM. RDoC advocates acknowledge that DSM categories have no solid foundation, but keep spreading the flawed idea that with the advent of the DSM-III diagnostic reliability increased: "This system [the DSM] has provided diagnostic reliability and descriptive utility, but has not led to satisfactory biological elaboration of the diagnostic constructs. Certainly, simple relationships between biological events and hypothesized diagnostic categories have not emerged. Also, more complex and subtle relationships between genetic and neural phenomena and mental illness have been elusive" (Kozak and Cuthbert 2016, p. 288).

A first important point of the RDoC project is that it aspires to develop a diagnostic framework that is not purely based on the description of syndromes, such that a step can be made from a focus on "mental disorders" toward "brain disorders" or "neural circuit disorders" (Insel and Cuthbert 2015, pp. 499–500). It is devoted to developing diagnostic categories that are not just conventional, but based on evidence of "underlying" illness dynamics: "the RDoC framework assumes that data from genetics and clinical neuroscience will yield biosignatures that will augment clinical symptoms and signs for clinical management" (Insel et al. 2010, p. 749). The idea of finding biosignatures expresses the belief that in the end research will reveal stable, measurable physical indicators of psychopathology, which in their turn will be useful reference points for reorganizing diagnostic categories. If such constant underlying referents are indeed found, the validity of psychiatric diagnoses would be greatly enhanced. Such a diagnostic system would break with the DSM as we know it since the DSM-III, in that pure conventional groupings of symptoms would not make up the basis of the system. This could in fact lead to a breakthrough in psychiatric thinking. However, the pragmatic objective of the RDoC initiative is far less focused on disorders, but consists of elaborating "a set of psychological constructs linked to behavioral dimensions for which strong evidence exists for circuits that implement these functions, and relate the extremes of functioning along these dimensions to specified symptoms (i.e., impairment)" (Kozak and Cuthbert 2016, p. 288). Doubts have been formulated as to whether this biopsychological focus on continuous dimensions of psychological functioning will actually yield clinically useful parameters. A key problem in this respect is the question as to how clinical cases might be discerned from ordinary distress: *"One of the striking omissions in the RDoC 'matrix' is* any appreciation of the remarkable difference between well and sick, or the critical importance of time in defining course or prognosis and in clinical decision-making. How one determines that somebody is a 'case' with disability and distress remains obscure, as there is no tactic, for example, to distinguish unhappiness or demoralization from clinical depression" (Weinberger et al. 2015, p. 1161). Indeed, many theorists of medicine and psychiatry have been stressing that psychopathology implies a qualitative break away from the experience of normality (Canguilhem 1966; Cooper 2007), which the RDoC project seems to ignore.

Specifically the RDoC project focuses on seven units of analysis: genes, molecules, cells, neural circuits, physiology (e.g., cortisol, heart rate), behavior, and self-report.[12] Behaviors and self-reports make up the descriptive level of the newly planned classification system, the five other levels concern different biological correlates. These units of analysis are applied to five broad domains of functioning, within which specific clinically relevant variables have been selected. The first domain is Negative Valence, and the core variables under investigation are acute threat (fear), potential threat (anxiety), sustained threat, frustrative non-reward (frustration), and loss. The second domain is Positive Valence, which includes approach motivation, initial responsiveness to reward, sustained responsiveness to reward, reward learning, and habit. Cognition makes

---

[12] See: http://www.nimh.nih.gov/research-priorities/rdoc/nimh-research-domain-criteria-rdoc.shtml

up the third domain the RDoC project investigates. Key variables under investigation are attention, perception, working memory, declarative memory, language, effortful cognitive control, and working memory. The fourth domain is Social Processes, with affiliation and attachment, social communication, self-perception and understanding, and other-perception and understanding as its key variables. The fifth domain is Arousal, and includes arousal as such (sensitivity to external and internal stimuli), circadian rhythms, and sleep/wakefulness. These domains and units of analysis have been formulated based on large panel discussions. Some believe that such consensus-based formulation again undermines the validity of future psychiatric diagnosis, and criticize the continued use of self-report (Weinberger et al. 2015). Indeed, a key problem with the RDoC matrix is that it is arbitrary in the domains and subdomains of functioning it discerns. For example, given the key importance of resilience and hope in the process of recovery from psychopathology, and of their counterparts in the formation of vulnerability for psychiatric symptoms, one might expect that such factors would be included in the RDoC matrix (Jeste et al. 2015). Yet this is not the case, and the reason why such positive mental health factors have been left aside is unclear. This might be an effect of the relative absence of a theoretical framework at the basis of formulating the matrix. Others point out that a key problem with the RDoC approach concerns its neglect of the test-retest reliability and stability of measurement methods used to examine specific cells of the RDoC matrix (Kraemer 2015).

However, a big question that remains open is whether the optimism about a pathophysiologically based diagnostic system that rests on the biopsychological examination of key psychological processes is realistic or not. The RDoC project breaks with the DSM in that it does not primarily focus on signs and symptoms of disorders. Rather, symptoms are seen as extreme outcomes of broad biopsychological processes that might be disturbed to certain degrees or not. Indeed, key to the project is its dimensional focus: disturbance is not conceptualized as categorical in nature, but as continuous, with various degrees of severity. Yet, will this eventually give rise to a pathophysiologically based diagnostic system?

The hope of finding such a pathophysiologically based diagnostic system is almost as old as modern psychiatry. Until now, this assumption has rarely produced evidence on strong associations between specific symptom profiles and biological markers, like specific genes or specific brain correlates that could be observed in an individual. Indeed, as Dennis Charney et al. (2002, p. 33) suggested in the DSM-5 research agenda: "the field of psychiatry has thus far failed to identify a single neurobiological phenotypic marker or gene that is useful in making a diagnosis of a major psychiatric disorder or for predicting response to psychopharmacologic treatment." They speculated that "it will be discovered that specific combinations of genes will relate to constellations of abnormalities in many brain-based functions—including but not limited to the regulation of mood, anxiety, perception, learning, memory, aggression, eating, sleeping, and sexual function—that will coalesce to form disease states heretofore unrecognized" (Charney et al. 2002, p. 71). This hope now seems to be reincarnated in the RDoC project. Interestingly, reasons usually mentioned for explaining why such system has not yet been developed again come down to *the technology alibi* that Berrios and Marková (2002) described: current research methods have helped us raise a corner of the veil, but in the near future better techniques will help us draw workable conclusions.

There is no doubt that with its biopsychological focus the RDoC project makes the dominant biomedical paradigm in contemporary psychiatry explicit, and that systematic investigation of this framework is certainly worthwhile. Examination of what the framework yields will elucidate its actual value and clarify whether this approach has important diagnostic and therapeutic implications. However, an interesting intermediate observation that Kozak and Cuthbert (2016) make is that when investigating specific constructs from one of the delineated domains—like fear—correlations between measures from different units of analysis—like genetics, neural circuits, behavior, and self-report—are usually modest: "Observed modest covariation among measures of fear across multiple units of analysis presents theoretical and practical *conundra*" (Kozak and Cuthbert 2016, p. 292). Often associations between different variables that are measured with the same instruments (e.g., self-report questionnaires) are stronger than associations between multiple measurements of single variables. Hence the following question: "How can one develop rules of inference for the presence of fear, or for that matter, any dimensional construct of psychopathology in the face of modest covariation in the very measures that must converge to validate a hypothesized construct?" (Kozak and Cuthbert 2016, p. 292). Most likely, RDoC-based research will give rise to *probabilistic thinking* about associations between units of analysis (e.g., genetics of fear versus self-reports about fear): depending on convergence of diverse measures, diagnostic certainty will increase. Importantly, this observation of modest covariations challenges the idea of "biosignatures" that Thomas Insel and colleagues (2010, p. 749) situated at the basis of the RDoC initiative. The idea of biosignatures suggests fixed relations between units of analysis, with stringent biological indicators at the basis of psychological variables. By contrast, the observed modest correlations between multiple measurements of single variables suggest that chance and uncertainty will have to be taken into account more strongly. Indeed, a main vulnerability of the RDoC initiative is that it might open up an era of biopsychological reification, in which psychological states are seen as mere indicators of underlying biological disturbances: "a search for biomarkers of RDoC constructs could also be subject to a misplaced desire for a 'gold standard'" (Kozak and Cuthbert 2016, p. 293).

This brings us to a second important point: the RDoC project builds only on research in biological psychiatry and experimentally oriented clinical psychology, thus neglecting other perspectives on psychopathology that stem from the social sciences and the humanities (see also Paris and Kirmayer 2016). Non-biomedical dimensions of human suffering are largely left out of consideration. Obviously, psychopathology has a biological component, yet it has many other facets as well, which the RDoC project, just as the DSM, neglects. In terms of the Cambridge Model of Symptom Formation, and the Triangular Model of Symptom Formation, the RDoC initiative has a limited focus: it concentrates on brain signals and related bodily processes, as well as on specific mental processes and symptoms, but it neglects all contextually based configuration processes and the embedment of symptoms in speech acts. Indeed, as it is completely focused on biological causation, the RDoC project doesn't take into account the fact that people are signifier-using creatures that have a reflexive relation to their own mental life and the world they live in, and that attempt to make sense of reality. In Foucauldian terms it might be concluded that such an approach bears witness to a *biopolitical* attitude toward human suffering (Kirshner 2009).

Most importantly, the RDoC project again seems to announce an approach to diagnosis in which a person's self-reflexive relation to his own suffering is neglected. The RDoC studies psychopathology only in a naturalizing way, taking psychopathology as an external object in the world that might only be grasped by neutral empirical description. It disregards how psychopathology makes up a structural way of relating to oneself and the world (or, in Lacanian terms, to the Real, the Symbolic, and the Imaginary), which determines the experience of subjectivity. For example, this is reflected in the strict parallelism between animal models of mental distress and research in humans within the RDoC initiative (see also Kirmayer and Crafa 2014). However, a fearful dog relates differently to his own fear than a human being. A fearful human does not simply undergo fear, but relates to it. We evaluate our fear in terms of normative beliefs and expectations, interpreting and situating the experienced state in terms of broader sets of ideas that are characteristic of who we are in terms of our life history, the socialization we had in our family, and multiple other social and cultural contexts.

In their account on the RDoC project, Kozak and Cuthbert (2016, p. 292) defend their approach by contrasting it with "subjectivism." What they call subjectivism comes down to the private ideas an individual holds about himself: "According to this tradition, subjective experience is the quintessential feature of an emotion, such as fear, and indicators such as behavior and physiology are taken to indicate this phenomenal state. This Cartesian dualism entails a logical conundrum: An oft-assumed inherent privacy of subjective experience renders it necessarily insusceptible to scientific measurement." In their view, the study of subjectivity seems restricted to gaining access to "phenomenal states" in the mind, that is, to getting hold of the contents of mental life through introspection. In a defense against such subjectivism they suggest that self-report only makes up one type of measurement, and that instead of introspection, the heterophenomenological approach formulated by Daniel Dennett (1991) should be taken into account more strongly: "Accordingly, experiential claims represent a kind of 'folk' psychology of the self that should be neither assumed veridical nor simply discounted"

(Kozak and Cuthbert 2016, p. 292). If the study of subjectivity implies such a romanticized focus on the irreducibility of private experiences, Kozak and Cuthbert's comment would make sense. Yet, phenomenological and psychoanalytical accounts of subjectivity typically have an entirely different focus, and also don't assume that a mere self-reflective introspective mapping of mental states provides veridical knowledge (Feyaerts and Vanheule 2015). The study of subjectivity is more concerned with *how* experience takes shape, *how* it is organized in mental states, and factors that determine these processes, than with mapping the flow of ideas and feelings occupying people's mind. For example, this can be seen in Husserl's (1950) emphasis on phenomenological reduction, which concentrates on how the experience of states and events is organized, or in the Lacanian study of the subject (Lacan 1964), which focuses on how the subject engaged in the speech act—the enunciating subject—differs from the subject as articulated in narratives—the enunciated subject. It can also be retraced in the Cambridge Model of Symptom Formation, which emphasizes the configuration processes along which symptom experience takes shape, and in our Triangular Model of Symptom Formation, which adds the systematic study of the speech act to the investigation of psychopathology. Taking into account subjectivity implies that symptoms and experiences are studied in the contexts in which they take shape. Consequently, the study of subjectivity cannot be reduced to the production of introspective self-report. Indeed, such inquiry does not shy away from systematic investigation, and does not imply a rejection of scientific examination, but typically assumes that examinations of how things are should also take into account the person for whom things are the way they are, and the world this person lives in.

Does this imply that the RDoC framework is entirely useless when considered from a subjectivity-oriented perspective? This is not necessarily the case. The five domains and respective subdomains from the RDoC matrix might indeed also be studied from contextual and subject-oriented points of view. For example, fear such as experienced in the instance of hallucinations might be explored systematically along such lines. Yet in doing so, theoretical and methodological paradigms should be used that diverge quite dramatically from the strictly quantifying and mainly experimentally based approach of the RDoC project.

The Mental Disorder: What Kind of Kind?

This reflection on the biopsychological focus of the RDoC initiative brings us to the question as to what mental disorders exactly are: should different disorders be thought of as species that have a status parallel to what biologists discern in the natural world? Or is such a claim overrated? And are the conventional labels invented by professionals over the years above all artificial? As already indicated in the previous section, the DSM seems to assume that mental disorders are *natural kinds*. The idea of natural kinds has a long-standing history in philosophy. As Rachel Cooper (2005, p. 46) indicates: "'Natural kind' is a technical term used by philosophers to refer to the kinds of thing or stuff studied by the natural sciences." H2O, bonobos, and birch trees[13] are examples of natural kinds: all have a fixed structure that can be discovered by means of empirical research, and they behave according to natural laws. Independent of what people think about these objects, and of how such objects are appreciated by humans, natural kinds function along fixed laws. Traditionally, the concept "natural kind" was used in contrast with "artificial kinds," which referred to artifacts of human work. However, some of these artifacts, like machines and lab-designed chemicals, also have a fixed structure, and behave according to stringent laws, which is why they cannot be simply separated. In his review of the "natural kind" concept, Ian Hacking (2006) indicates that so many contradicting claims about natural kinds circulate in literature that the concept itself has self-destructed. He indicates that "kinds," which are things, states, or events that we call with the same name (e.g., " trees," "dogs," "depression"), are always distinguished by classifying human beings, and that the degree to which these are natural or not is variable. Discussions about natural kinds started in the Victorian era, when scientists were highly concerned with classifying the many objects they discovered (plants, animals, stones, etc.) in taxonomies. Typically, at first taxonomies are seen as artificial and pragmatically useful grouping schemes. Yet, as time evolves such schemes are often taken

---

[13] In psychology, different emotions, like happiness, sadness, anger and anxiety, are sometimes considered as natural kinds. However, whether this is justified or not remains an object of continuous debate (Lindquist et al. 2013).

as reflections of nature itself, which illustrates our common tendency toward reifying interpretation. Hacking argues that qualifying kinds as "natural" or not is illusory. Indeed, each classification reflects choices and preferences. The degree to which a kind is natural depends on our natural scientific insight in the phenomenon under study. Therefore, in line with William Whewell, he defends the following characterization, which above all stresses the pragmatic value, logical coherence, and empirical correctness of classifications: "a kind is a class denoted by a common name about which there is the possibility of general, intelligible and consistent, and probably true assertions" (Hacking 2006, p. 34).

No matter how abstract the question as to whether mental disorders are natural kinds might be, it is an issue with direct impact since it defines the public and scientific status of psychiatry. Indeed, often the adjective "natural" is taken as a quality label that is presumed to define the public and scientific status of the kind one is interested in: "If mental disorders are natural kinds then there will be laws, explanations and sound inductive inferences in psychiatry—in short psychiatry will be a genuine science. If on the other hand mental disorders are not natural kinds, whether psychiatry is a science must be questioned" (Cooper 2005, p. 46). As discussed in Chap. 2, in the 1970s critical scholars questioned the scientific status of psychiatry and by pointing to *labeling* and *reification* they cast serious doubts on the so-called *natural kind* status of mental disorders. They paid the price of being damned and extradited by the psychiatric establishment and were eventually overruled by the neo-Kraepelinian restoration movement.

Indeed, the issue of *the kind of thing a mental disorder is* needs to be approached carefully. As a first possibility, mental disorders might be thought of as *essentialist kinds*. Within this view, mental disorders are indeed natural kinds and a single underlying reality is presumed to be at the basis of each disorder. Disorders then differ in that they obey different natural laws and they exist in reality regardless of whether we detected them or not: "essentialist kinds have essences, and they exist whether or not we recognize them" (Kendler et al. 2011, p. 1144). Essentialist accounts of natural kinds assume that well-defined biological etiologic disturbances are to be found at the basis of mental disorders, like specific deficiencies in the brain or genetic defects. The roots of such essentialist disorder accounts can be found in anatomo-pathological explanations of disease. In 1822, the French physician Antoine Laurent Bayle described the disease of *general paralysis*. Qua syndrome, general paralysis is characterized by delusions that normally start with exaltation. Throughout the years these fade out; the individual ends up with deterioration, amnesia, and dementia. Bayle argued that general paralysis results from a chronic inflammation of the brain. Later on, in 1913, the Japanese bacteriologist Hideyo Noguchi demonstrated that the bacterium that causes syphilis (*Treponema pallidum*) affected the brain tissues of paralytic dementia patients. Moreover, 30 years later penicillin proved to be an effective medicine for treating the *Treponema pallidum* bacteria, and the once prevalent neurosyphilis quickly became a rare disease. This discovery was idealized, fueling the belief that similar unequivocal essences could be found at the basis of all mental disorders. However, what was obfuscated by this idealization was the fact that only a limited number of untreated syphilitic patients actually develop general paralysis, meaning that the actual cause of neurosyphilis is not as straightforward as the essentialists might have hoped (Verhaeghe 2002).

Nowadays, such essentialist accounts are considered naïve: "In the 19th and early 20th centuries, the successful demonstration of a single infectious etiology for general paresis of the insane led to the idea that single, discrete causes might exist for other major psychiatric disorders. Over a century of increasingly sophisticated neurobiological research has failed to fulfill this vision" (Kendler et al. 2011, p. 1144). For example, contrary to what was first hoped, genes are no longer considered to be such candidate essences: "no genetic marker has yet been shown to be useful in prospectively identifying any specific psychiatric disorder" (Dubovsky 2016, p. 130; see also McNally 2011). Nonetheless, the tendency to essentialize mental disorders is deeply ingrained in the lines of reasoning of both laymen and professionals (Adriaens and De Block 2013). Indeed, the DSM-5 also seems to flirt with such a naïve essentialist view of mental disorders. This is reflected in the claim that the DSM-5 aimed "to carve nature at its joints" (Regier et al. 2009, p. 648). The idea of "joints in nature" suggests that the world of psychopathology contains a well-defined fixed internal structure that simply awaits scientific discovery. Such a view bears witness to an essentialist model of mental disorders (Kendler et al. 2011; Lilienfeld and Marino 1999). The idea that "diagnoses in the DSM-III, DSM-III-R, and DSM-IV are best understood as useful *placeholders*" (Bernstein 2011, my italics) while the DSM-5 provides us with validated alternatives also bears witness to naïve essentialism. The idea of the placeholder suggests that one day the "real category" will replace the artificial label. Given the fact that the DSM-5 doesn't differ much from its predecessors, one cannot but conclude that the manual attempts to keep the essentialist dream alive, while in actual fact it by no means lives up to the standard it aspires for.

In contrast with essentialist *natural kind* accounts, forms of psychopathology could also be thought of as *practical kinds* (Zachar 2002). Resting on the philosophical ground of pragmatism, the practical kind account assumes that no unambiguous reality can be found in the world that simply awaits discovery. Indeed, several valuable ways of cutting the world up could be designed, albeit some classifications have better practical implications than others and hence should be favored. As Peter Zachar (2002, p. 219) indicates: "The practical kinds model does not deny that things have internal structures; it only denies that internal structure by itself determines category membership." What really matters in terms of developing pragmatic classification systems is what one can *do* with them. For example, in Zachar's view classifications are good if constituent categories are clinically useful; can be effectively linked to potential treatment modalities; can aid experimental research; cohere with basic science, like genetics, physiology, and psychology; and ultimately give rise to reliable diagnoses. In such a view, validity is a quality that needs to be demonstrated through clinical practice and research, not an inherent feature presumed to be at the basis of mental disorders, as is characteristic of the essentialist perspective.

Despite the scientific aspirations of the DSM-5, it seems that, at best, DSM disorders could be thought of as practical kinds. This means that laypeople and scientists alike should not simply assume that they are caused by biological disturbances. On the contrary, clear-cut biological disturbances prove to be related to only a few psychiatric disorders. Interestingly, while critical researchers have long pointed to problems with the pragmatic value of the DSM, biological researchers now draw attention to its limits as well. Hyman (2010), for example, indicates that the DSM categories don't map with the biological structures underlying psychopathology and suggests that research designs formulated in terms of DSM categories *hinder scientific progress*. More recently, Thomas Insel (2013; Kapur et al. 2012), the director of the US NIMH when the DSM-5 was published, suggested that most diagnostic categories in the DSM don't connect with underlying biological structures, hence his call for research that crosses DSM categories. Indeed, the RDoC project of the NIMH made such a step and studies biological structures and mental symptoms irrespective of the various disorder categories outlined in the DSM (Insel et al. 2010).

Apparently, the RDoC project continues to assume that mental disorders are natural kinds. Its exclusive focus on biological determinants of mental symptoms bears witness of this naturalistic attitude. However, the approach taken there leaves aside essentialist interpretations, and paves the way for more flexible natural kind accounts of mental disorders. An important example of a more flexible natural kind account can be found in the work of Kendler et al. (2011, p. 1146), who suggest that mental disorders might be seen as "mechanistic property clusters" (MPC). In their view, the practical kind approach is not sufficiently etiological or explanatory in nature. They believe that disorders are not merely pragmatic groupings of mental symptoms and suggest that there are "robust explanatory structures to be discovered underlying most psychiatric disorders" (Kendler et al. 2011, p. 1146). At the same time they don't buy into the essentialist kind account: "The 'kindness' of species is not, from an MPC perspective, produced by a defining essence but rather from more or less stable patterns of complex interaction between behavior, environment and physiology that have arisen through development, evolution and interaction with an environment" (Kendler et al. 2011, pp. 1146–1147). In their view, psychiatric patients' illness conditions reflect a limited number of mind/brain states, which basic research should discover. A similar account can be found in the work of Rachel Cooper (2005, 2007). In her view, mental disorders make up natural kinds since they have similar *determining properties*: "as the determining properties of members of a natural kind are similar, so long as environmental factors are kept constant, members of a natural kind end up being similar in many respects" (Cooper 2005, p. 51). She argues that mental disorders are natural kinds to the extent that they obey the same natural laws; disorders are not physical entities "present in the Garden of Eden," but conditions that behave similarly in similar environments (Cooper 2005, p. 52).

What is key to these "natural kind" perspectives is that they all start from a philosophically realist and (post-)positivist perspective: human characteristics, like mental disorders, are empirical objects that must be studied with the experimental method of the natural sciences, which is thus valued as a superior method for gaining knowledge. What these explanations don't take into account is the notion of the human being qua self-reflexive transcendental subject living in specific contexts. Indeed, mental disorders are not neutral objects, but mind/body states people actively manipulate through symbolic activity. Consequently, the study of psychopathology is partial when it neglects the way we relate to our mental reality. Moreover, people are not just plants living in an "environment": they actively manipulate and create mental, social, and cultural contexts, and, moreover, generate meaning about them, which can change over time. Thus considered, Ian Hacking (2002) was correct when he wittily argued that mental disorders are above all *human kinds*: products of human activity that are directed toward control and social recognition. Diagnoses carry meaning—some are desirable, others not at all—and affect and change those who are classified. For example, based on disorder labels people create advocacy groups and construct identities, which contain do's and don'ts for "true" specimens of that kind.

Therefore, instead of using static *natural kind* accounts of psychopathology we should perhaps consider psychopathology in terms of *reflexive kinds*. By holding on to the idea of "kinds," we on the one hand suggest that, indeed, psychopathology may be governed by laws and structures that can be described in scientific terms, yet a proper study of psychopathology requires more than just a biomedical focus. On the other hand, these laws do not apply to the cases we meet in the clinic unequivocally. Indeed, in clinical contexts we don't meet disorders or kinds of psychopathology, but people in whose life mental health problems take shape, and who might be qualified as a case or not. As one studies specific cases, particularities as well as singularities will be discerned: next to generalizable characteristics, psychiatric problems always have context-specific and case-specific qualities. Indeed, the reflexive relation humans have to their own mind/body states implies that they cannot be wholly generalized across cases. This is not a problem, but it requires a *casuistic approach* to diagnosis that doesn't merely determine which type of psychopathology applies to a given person. Diagnoses should also describe and document *how* and *to what extent* such a *patterned* way of functioning can be discerned. Next to that, diagnosis should describe how psychopathology is related to *idiosyncratic* events and to the way in which the person deals with such events. In doing so, special attention should be paid to singularity, as discussed earlier in this chapter. From a Lacanian point of view this, above all, implies that the dimension of *the subject* and the individual's way of being confronted with *the Real* should be taken into account. Indeed, contra the neo-Kraepelian doxa I believe that diagnosis is more than classification. It consists of mapping the regularities, irregularities, and deadlocks in a person's functioning and of grasping contextual factors that determine the way in which a person tries to make sense of his own distress.

Conclusion

Etymologically, the term "diagnosis" means "to distinguish," and "to know thoroughly." In the DSM all attention goes to the component of distinguishing, where it is assumed that all cases with the same disorder will obey the same natural laws. Taking the epistemological status of mental symptoms into account, this is unjustifiable. In clinical practice one doesn't meet specimens of diagnostic manuals, but contextualized cases that can never be fully grasped by classifications, hence the *reflexive kinds* account of psychopathology.

Based on my previous arguments, I conclude that the DSM (from the DSM-III until the DSM-5) uses a naïve medical semiotic model: symptoms are signs of underlying conditions that can be studied independently from their context. In this view, context variables only play a moderating role that might alter the shape of mental symptoms, but don't determine the core characteristics of the symptom. Associated with this point of view, the DSM starts from the assumption that, essentially, mental disorders are neurobiological natural kinds. This viewpoint makes up a rhetoric discursive position that feeds the credibility of psychiatric diagnosis, yet this position remains unproven: unambiguous non-overlapping biological validators have never been successfully connected to any of the DSM categories. By concentrating on "biopsychopathology" and "biopsychological" research only, the RDoC project of the NIMH again seems to take such a naturalizing focus, which neglects the self-reference that people have when they experience distress, as well as the contextual embedment of mental health problems.

In contrast with the decontextualizing DSM approach, I believe that mental symptoms should above all be studied within relevant contexts. Obviously, the biology of the body is an important context within which symptoms arise. Yet there are many other contexts that cannot be neglected and should be taken into account in making a diagnosis. Humans should not only be seen as objects that are suitable for naturalistic examination, but also as signifier-using creatures that keep track of their own lives and have memories and experiences in which symptoms are embedded. What is more, human subjects relate to one another, live in social contexts, and thrive on cultural determinants.

Obviously, the project of taking into account context confronts psychiatric diagnosis with new problems that haven't been addressed in this chapter. A contextualizing approach is especially relevant for studying symptoms, but might be challenging if one solely aims to group symptoms into syndromes (Marková and Berrios 2009). However, this should not necessarily be the case. In line with my discussion of Lacan's theory of clinical structures, it is justified to presume that a contextualizing approach might cohere with the project of discerning relevant subtypes of psychopathology for which different treatment approaches are needed.

Other References

Adriaens, P., & De Block, A. (2013). Why we essentialize mental disorders. *Journal of Medicine and Philosophy, 38*, 107–127.

Andreasen, N. (2001). Diversity in psychiatry: Or, why did we become psychiatrists? *American Journal of Psychiatry, 158*, 673–675.

Beavan, V., Read, J., & Cartwright, C. (2011). The prevalence of voice-hearers in the general population: A literature review. *Journal of Mental Health, 20*, 281–292.

Bernstein, C. A. (2011). Meta-structure in DSM-5 process. *Psychiatric News, 46*(5), 7–29.

Berrios, G. E. (1999). Classifications in psychiatry: A conceptual history. *Australian and New Zealand Journal of Psychiatry, 33*, 145–160.

Berrios, G. E. (2012). The 19th-century nosology of alienism: History and epistemology. In K. S. Kendler & J. Parnas (Eds.), *Philosophical issues in psychiatry II – Nosology* (pp. 101–117). Oxford: Oxford University Press.

Berrios, G. E., & Marková, I. S. (2002). Conceptual issues. In H. D'haenen, J. A. den Boer, & P. Willner (Eds.), *Biological psychiatry* (pp. 9–39). Chichester: Wiley.

Berrios, G. E., & Marková, I. S. (2006). Symptoms: Historical perspective and effect on diagnosis. In M. Blumenfield & J. J. Strain (Eds.), *Psychosomatic medicine* (pp. 27–38). Philadelphia: Lippincott Williams & Wilkins.

Bird, A., & Tobin, E. (2010). Natural kinds. In E. N. Zalta (Ed.), *The Stanford encyclopedia of philosophy (Summer 2010 edition)*. Retrieved September 16, 2011, from http://plato.stanford.edu/archives/sum2010/entries/natural-kinds/.

Borsboom, D., & Cramer, A. O. J. (2013). Network analysis: An integrative approach to the structure of psychopathology. *Annual Review of Clinical Psychology, 9*, 91–121.

Boschloo, L., van Borkulo, C. D., Rhemtulla, M., Keyes, K. M., Borsboom, D., & Schoevers, R. A. (2015). The network structure of symptoms of the diagnostic and statistical manual of mental disorders. *PLoS ONE, 10*, e0137621.

Bracken, P., Thomas, P., Timimi, S., et al. (2012). Psychiatry beyond the current paradigm. *British Journal of Psychiatry, 201*, 430–434.

Buchheim, A., Viviani, R., Kessler, H., et al. (2013). Changes in prefrontal-limbic function in major depression after 15 months of long-term psychotherapy. *Plos One, 7*, e33745.

Canguilhem, G. (1966). *The normal and the pathological*. Brooklyn: Zone Books.

Charney, D. S., Barlow, D. H., Botteron, K., et al. (2002). Neuroscience research agenda to guide development of a pathophysiologically based classification system. In D. J. Kupfer, M. B. First, & D. A. Regier (Eds.), *A research agenda for DSM-V* (pp. 31–83). Washington, DC: American Psychiatric Association.

Cooper, R. (2005). *Classifying madness – A philosophical examination of the diagnostic and statistical manual of mental disorders*. Dordrecht: Springer.

Cooper, R. (2007). *Psychiatry and philosophy of science*. Stocksfield: Acumen.
Dar-Nimrod, I., & Heine, S. J. (2011). Genetic essentialism: On the deceptive determinism of DNA. *Psychological Bulletin, 137*, 800–818.
de Saussure, F. (1916). *Course in general linguistics*. New York: Philosophical Library.
De Vos, J. (2014). Which materialism? Questioning the matrix of psychology, neurology, psychoanalysis and ideology critique. *Theory and Psychology, 24,* 76–92.
Decker, H. (2013). *The making of DSM-III*. New York: Oxford University Press.
Dennett, D. C. (1991). *Consciousness explained*. Boston: Little Brown.
Dubovsky, S. L. (2016). The limitations of genetic testing in psychiatry. *Psychotherapy and Psychosomatics, 85*, 129–135.
Eco, U. (1976). *A theory of semiotics*. London: Macmillan.
Evrard, R. (2013). Psychopathology and exceptional experiences: A literature review. *L'Évolution Psychiatrique, 78*, 155–176.
Feyaerts, J., & Vanheule, S. (2015). How to return to subjectivity? Natorp, Husserl and Lacan on the limits of reflection. *Theory & Psychology, 25*, 753–774.
Frances, A. (2013). *Saving normal – An insider's revolt against out-of-control psychiatric diagnosis, DSM-5, big pharma, and the medicalization of ordinary life*. New York: William Morrow & Harper Collins Publishers.
Freud, S. (1953 [1913]). On beginning the treatment (Further recommendations on the technique of psychoanalysis I). In *The standard edition of the complete psychological works for Sigmund Freud* (Vol. 12, pp. 121–144). London: Hogarth Press.
Good, B. J. (1994). *Medicine, rationality, and experience. An anthropological perspective*. Cambridge: Cambridge University Press.
Hacking, I. (2002). Inaugural lecture: Chair of philosophy and history of science concepts at the Collège de France, 16 January 2001. *Economy and Society, 31*, 1–14.
Husserl, E. (1950). *Cartesian meditations*. Dordrecht: Kluwer Academic Publishers.
Hyman, S. E. (2010). The diagnosis of mental disorders: The problem of reification. *Annual Review of Clinical Psychology, 6*, 155–179.
Insel, T. (2013). Transforming diagnosis. *Blogpost*. Retrieved December 10, 2013, from http://www.nimh.nih.gov/about/director/2013/transforming-diagnosis.shtml.
Insel, T., & Cuthbert, B. (2015). Brain disorders? Precisely. *Science, 348*, 499–500.

Insel, T. & Lieberman, J.A. (2013). DSM-5 and RDoC: Shared interests. *Blogpost*. Retrieved December 11, 2013, from http://www.nimh.nih.gov/news/science-news/2013/dsm-5-and-rdoc-shared-interests.shtml.

Insel, T., Cuthbert, B., Garvey, M., Heinssen, R., Pine, D.S.n., Quinn, K., Sanislow, C., & Wang, P. (2010). Research Domain Criteria (RDoC): Toward a new classification framework for research on mental disorders. *American Journal of Psychiatry, 167*, 748–751.

Jeste, D. V., Palmer, B. W., Rettew, D. C., & Boardman, S. (2015). Positive psychiatry: Its time has come. *Journal of Clinical Psychiatry, 76*, 675–683.

Kagan, J. (2012). *Psychology's ghosts – The crisis in the profession and the way back*. New Haven/London: Yale University Press.

Kapur, S., Phillips, A. G., & Insel, T. R. (2012). Why has it taken so long for biological psychiatry to develop clinical tests and what to do about it? *Molecular Psychiatry, 17*, 1174–1179.

Karlsson, H. (2011). How psychotherapy changes the brain. *Psychiatric Times, 28*. Retrieved November 12, 2013, from http://www.psychiatrictimes.com/psychotherapy/how-psychotherapy-changes-brain.

Keim Campbell, J., O'Rourke, M., & Slater, M. H. (2011). *Carving nature at its joints: Natural kinds in metaphysics and science*. Cambridge: MIT Press.

Kelleher, I., Jenner, J., & Cannon, M. (2010). Psychotic symptoms in the general population – An evolutionary perspective. *British Journal of Psychiatry, 197*, 167–169.

Kendler, K. S., Zachar, P., & Craver, C. (2011). What kinds of things are psychiatric disorders? *Psychological Medicine, 41*, 1143–1150.

Kirmayer, L. J., & Crafa, D. (2014). What kind of science for psychiatry. *Frontiers in Human Neuroscience, 8*, 435.

Kirshner, L. (2009). Biopolitics and the transformation of the psychiatric subject. In S. Binkley & J. Capetillo (Eds.), *A Foucault for the 21st century: Governmentality, biopolitics and discipline in the new millennium* (pp. 92–104). Newcastle upon Tyne: Cambridge Scholars Publishing.

Kozak, M. J., & Cuthbert, B. N. (2016). The NIMH research domain criteria initiative: Background, issues and pragmatics. *Psychophysiology, 53*, 286–297.

Kraemer, H. C. (2015). Research Domain Criteria (RDoC) and the DSM – Two methodological approaches to mental health diagnosis. *JAMA Psychiatry, 72*, 1163–1164.

Kupfer, D. J., & Regier, D. A. (2011). Neuroscience, clinical evidence, and the future of psychiatric classification in DSM-5. *American Journal of Psychiatry, 168*, 672–674.

Kupfer, D. J., First, M. B., & Regier, D. A. (2002). *A research agenda for DSM-V*. Washington, DC: American Psychiatric Association.

Lacan, J. (1964). *The seminar 1964, book XI, the four fundamental concepts of psycho-analysis*. London/New York: Karnac.

Lacan, J. (2006 [1947]). Presentation on psychical causality. In J. Lacan & J. A. Miller (Eds.), *Écrits* (pp. 123–158). New York/London: W. W. Norton.

Lacan, J. (2006 [1957]). The instance of the letter in the unconscious or reason since Freud. In J. Lacan & J. A. Miller (Eds.), *Écrits* (pp. 412–442). New York/London: W. W. Norton.

Lacan, J. (2006 [1959]). On a question prior to any possible treatment of psychosis. In J. Lacan & J. A. Miller (Eds.), *Écrits* (pp. 445–488). New York/London: W. W. Norton.

Lilienfeld, S. O., & Marino, L. (1999). Essentialism revisited: Evolutionary theory and the concept of mental disorder. *Journal of Abnormal Psychology, 108*, 400–411.

Lindquist, K. A., Siegel, E. H., Quigley, K. S., & Battett, L. F. (2013). The hundred-year emotion way: Are emotions natural kinds or psychological constructions? Comment on Lench, Flores, and Bench (2011). *Psychological Bulletin, 139*, 255–263.

Marková, I. S., & Berrios, G. E. (2009). Epistemology of mental symptoms. *Psychopathology, 42*, 343–349.

McNally, R. J. (2011). *What is mental illness?* Cambridge/London: Belknap Harvard.

Moore, J. (2001). On distinguishing methodological from radical behaviorism. *European Journal of Behavioral Analysis, 2*, 221–244.

Nobus, D. (2000). *Jacques Lacan and the Freudian practice of psychoanalysis*. New York: Routledge.

Paris, J., & Kirmayer, L. J. (2016). The national institute of mental health research domain criteria: A bridge too far. *Journal of Nervous and Mental Disease, 204*, 26–32.

Parker, I. (2010). *Lacanian psychoanalysis – Revolutions on subjectivity*. London/New York: Routledge.

Parnas, J. (2012). The nature of the psychiatric object and classification. In K. S. Kendler & J. Parnas (Eds.), *Philosophical issues in psychiatry II – nosology* (pp. 118–123). Oxford: Oxford University Press.

Pechey, R., & Halligan, P. (2011). The prevalence of delusion-like beliefs relative to sociocultural beliefs in the general population. *Psychopathology, 44*, 106–115.
Pechey, R., & Halligan, P. (2012). Prevalence and correlates of anomalous experiences in a large non-clinical sample. *Psychology and Psychotherapy: Theory, Research and Practice, 85*, 150–162.
Regier, D. A., Narrow, W. E., Kuhl, E. A., & Kupfer, D. J. (2009). The conceptual development of DSM-V. *American Journal of Psychiatry, 166*, 645–650.
Reynolds, C. F., Lewis, D. A., Detre, T., Schatzberg, A. F., & Kupfer, D. J. (2009). The future of psychiatry as clinical neuroscience. *Academic Medicine, 84*, 446–450.
Rose, N. (1996). *Inventing our selves – Psychology, power and personhood*. Cambridge: Cambridge University Press.
Rose, N. (1999). *Governing the soul – The shaping of the private self – Second edition*. London/New York: Free Association Books.
Sandifer, M. S., Hordern, A., & Green, L. M. (1970). The psychiatric interview: The impact of the first three minutes. *American Journal of Psychiatry, 126*, 968–973.
Stein, D. J., Phillips, K. A., Bolton, D., Fulford, K. W. M., Sadler, J. S., & Kendler, K. S. (2010). What is a mental/psychiatric disorder? From DSM-IV to DSM-V. *Psychological Medicine, 40*, 1759–1765.
Stoyanov, D., Machamer, P. K., Schaffner, K. F., & Rivera-Hernández, R. (2012). The challenge of psychiatric nosology and diagnosis. *Journal of Evaluation in Clinical Practice, 18*, 704–709.
Trudgen, R. (2000). *Why warriors lie down and die. Towards an understanding of why the Aboriginal people of Arnhem land face the greatest crisis in health and education since European contact*. Darwin: Aboriginal Resource and Developmental Services Inc.
Van Os, J. (2010). Are psychiatric diagnoses of psychosis scientific and useful? The case of schizophrenia. *Journal of Mental Health, 19*, 305–317.
Van Os, J. (2016). "Schizophrenia" does not exist. *The British Medical Journal, 352*, i375.
Vanheule, S. (2011). *The subject of psychosis – A Lacanian perspective*. London/New York: Palgrave MacMillan.
Vanheule, S. (2012). Diagnosis in the field of psychotherapy: A plea for an alternative to the DSM-5.x. *Psychology and Psychotherapy: Theory, Research and Practice, 85*, 128–142.

Verhaeghe, P. (2002). *On being normal and other disorders*. New York: Other Press.

Verhaeghe, P. (2014). *What about me? – The struggle for identity in a market-based society*. Victoria/London: Scribe.

Watters, E. (2010). *Crazy like us: The globalization of the American psyche*. New York: Free Press.

Weinberger, D. R., Glick, I. D., & Klein, D. F. (2015). Whither Research Domain Criteria (RDoC)? The good, the bad, and the ugly. *JAMA Psychiatry, 72*, 1161–1162.

Westen, D. (2012). Protoype diagnosis of psychiatric syndromes. *World Psychiatry, 11*, 16–21.

Wilkinson, R. G., & Pickett, L. (2009). *The spirit level: Why more equal societies almost always do better*. London: Allan Lane.

Zachar, P. (2002). The practical kinds model as a pragmatist theory of classification. *Philosophy, Psychology and Psychiatry, 9*, 219–227.

4

From Mental Suffering to Mental Disorder and Back Again

What Do We Diagnose?

When exactly is a thought, feeling, or behavior disturbed, and does it bear witness to psychopathology, or to a mental disorder? The question is simple, but the answer is far less so. Evidently, upon making diagnoses, we make decisions about specific actions and interactions. For example, this is most clear in the DSM, with its checklists of disorder criteria that need to be evaluated. Take the diagnosis of ADHD; the first criterion listed for the aspect of inattention is the following: "Often fails to give close attention to details or makes careless mistakes in schoolwork, at work, or during other activities (e.g., overlooks or misses details, work is inaccurate)," and the last one in the list is: "Is often forgetful in daily activities (e.g., doing chores, running errands; for older adolescents and adults, returning calls, paying bills, keeping appointments)" (DSM-5, p. 59). What is remarkable about these criteria is that they are worded in ambiguous language, which implies that they leave much space for interpretation and appreciation. For example, when are mistakes in classwork "careless" in nature? Or at what point is "forgetfulness" in daily life abnormal?

The following clinical situation can illustrate the difficulty. One day a mother consulted me about her son. His primary school teacher is very unhappy with how he functions at school, and suggests to the mother that medication for ADHD might solve the problem. The mother is also concerned about her son. The boy is often careless while completing assignments, and forgetfulness is another problem. On several occasions he has forgotten his lunch box at school; his sports bag has also gone missing. Yet, are these behaviors a reason for major concern and do they make up a legitimate cause for medical intervention? According to the teacher, who is displeased with the boy's functioning, they are. However, the mother is hesitant. The boy, in his turn, experiences unease at school, yet his concerns particularly concern the teacher's brutal style of interaction in the classroom, which the mother recognizes. The child has difficulty with reading and spelling, which irritates the teacher. Personally, I conclude that the boy's apparent carelessness actually reflects his difficulty with spelling and reading, as well as a certain clash between the teacher's approach and the boy's spontaneous style of interaction. The boy's forgetfulness seems to be related to the overall unease he experiences in the school, where the teacher holds fast to a psychiatrizing focus.

This example illustrates major issues in diagnostic decision-making: which criteria really matter in evaluating a situation of distress? Whose opinions are the most important in evaluating specific mental states or behaviors? And based on which norms can one legitimately judge whether an individual's functioning makes up a source for major concern or not?

In the DSM these questions are not raised, nor does the handbook encourage clinicians to dwell on such issues, ethically reflect on how diagnostic judgments are best made, or how such judgments should be substantiated in terms of what is morally at stake when an individual's behavior is evaluated. Yet these questions matter. As Eric Parens and Josephine Johnston (2011) indicate in a Hastings Center special report, diagnoses are rooted in evaluations, which are always value-laden. Indeed, when both formulating and implementing diagnostic criteria and guidelines, value judgments and subjective opinions about what is normal or not determine our actions: "The exact boundaries between, for example, healthy and unhealthy anxiety or healthy and unhealthy aggression are

4 From Mental Suffering to Mental Disorder and Back Again   135

not written in nature; they are articulated by human beings living and working in particular places and times" (Parens and Johnston 2011, p. 4). Given the central impact of ethical values, great care needs to be taken with respect to whose opinions predominate in diagnostic judgment about what is acceptable and what is normal.

From a Lacanian point of view it might be argued that diagnostic situations should above all start from emptiness at the level of moral expectations, or from an "ethics of the lack." This does not mean that ethical stakes should be ignored, but that diagnosticians should by no means take any morally based criterion for granted in judging an individual's functioning. The main task for the diagnostician consists of noting and addressing the suffering or distress the patient expresses, without taking for granted what signs of distress actually mean, or judging whether behaviors are acceptable or not. The "good" that the diagnostician should above all engage in is *good listening*, and considering what the patient is expressing.

In his seminar on ethics Lacan (1959–1960) discusses the necessity of an ethics of the lack via the provocative example of Saint Martin of Tours. As a young man Saint Martin, who lived in the fourth century AD, was a soldier of the Roman army in Gaul. According to the legend, Martin of Tours, the soldier, met a naked beggar at one of the gates of the city of Amiens and gave him half of his cloak. Since he was a Roman soldier half of the cloak was owned by the Roman Empire, meaning that he gave away the part he owned himself. The following night Martin of Tours dreamt that Christ was wearing the half-cloak he had given away, and that their interaction in fact actualized one of the seven Works of Mercy from Christian religion: to clothe the naked. This story might be read as an exploit: the wealthy Martin of Tours pitifully shares with a poor beggar, thus exemplifying what a good man should do. Lacan's reading is somewhat different, and stresses that above all Martin of Tours made a major supposition that what the naked beggar needed was clothing. According to Lacan nothing guarantees that this supposition was correct. Indeed, "We are no doubt touching a primitive requirement in the need to be satisfied there, for the beggar is naked. But perhaps over and above that need to be clothed, he was begging for something else, namely, that Saint Martin either kill him or fuck him"

(Lacan 1959–1960, p. 186). The presumption that Martin of Tours made covers the beggar's perspective, hiding it way under the cloak of charity, thus precluding that the otherness of the other can be expressed. Martin of Tours fails to get hold of the element that doesn't fit within the framework he takes for granted. Without explicitly addressing the other's disarray, he assumes that he knows what is good for the beggar. Thus, the benefactor not only imposes normative interpretations and values onto the other, but also receives narcissistic gratification: his cloak is ruined, but the good is at his side. This installs a power relation, which grants a superior position to the benefactor. Yet, the beggar might refuse to comply with the evolving scenario. No doubt such an attitude would provoke outrage in the benefactor, which is exactly why the diagnostician does better when engaging in good listening instead of offering the good he possesses.

Indeed, when making diagnoses, an individual's mental and social functioning is evaluated. Careful diagnosis requires that the diagnostician act thoughtfully when judging specific behaviors and mental states. Usually, diagnosis evaluates whether someone's functioning bears witness to *psychopathology*, *abnormality*, or *mental disorder*. Psychopathology, abnormality, and mental disorder are the attributes that a diagnosis maps. These three concepts should not be thought of a synonymous. In the next sections I discuss the dissimilarity between these concepts, arguing that someone's experience of *pathos* should guide clinical diagnostic decision-making. Indeed, clinical diagnosis should not be so much concerned with detecting abnormalities or catching mental disorders, but above all with getting hold of psychopathology.

Psychopathology

Etymologically, the concept psychopathology is rooted in the word "pathos," which stems from the old Greek word "paschein," and refers to suffering. Psychopathology implies an experience of distress that disturbs an individual's functioning. Indeed, only if a person suffers from the way (s)he functions mentally, and significant mental pain can be observed, can a problem be qualified as "clinical" or "pathological" in nature. In her philosophical reflections on the object of psychiatry, Rachel Cooper (2005) epitomizes this by stating that in order to qualify a mental state as pathological or diseased, three conditions must be fulfilled: the individual should experience her mental state as something that is bad, she should be agonized by what she lives through and therefore be unhappy, and her mental state should be treatable.

The first condition stresses that an individual's way of functioning is only diseased if one feels the victim of what one is living through. Some people hear voices and are tormented by what they perceive. Others experience similar phenomena, but are not hindered or even feel fine with the extraordinary perceptions they have (see: Laroi 2012). In the first group the experience of excessive burden makes up a reason for diagnosis, which is lacking in the second case. Cooper (2005, p. 26) articulates this as follows: "Here I am suggesting that we should think about diseases in a way analogous to the way in which we think about weeds. A plant is only a weed if it is not wanted. Thus a daisy can be a weed in one garden but a flower in another, depending on whether or not it is a good thing in a particular garden." Indeed, following this line of reasoning, an individual hearing voices, who rarely feels disturbed by what she hears, bears witness to a remarkable psychological phenomenon that deviates from population norms, but cannot be considered a clinical case.

Cooper's (2005) second criterion stresses that a clinical diagnosis of disease can only be made if a person suffers and is unlucky because of the peculiarities experienced in her own functioning. People suffer if they can remember or imagine a life in which certain unwanted aspects of functioning were not present. When such an aspiration of an ideal self-image that is freed from the negative condition one currently bears witness to is missing, clinicians should give no diagnosis.

The third criterion Cooper (2005) adds to the list is that a diagnosis of psychiatric disease can only be made if the condition a person suffers from is amenable to psychiatric treatment. This characteristic, which Cooper seems to interpret in a far too medical way, enables us to distinguish between mental health problems and other conditions. For example, poverty might also be considered as an agonizing condition people suffer from. Yet, it is not a situation that should be diagnosed, because psychological and psychiatric interventions cannot solve the problem, while poverty-oriented interventions and societal changes might have beneficial effect. Obviously, the lack of money might come hand in hand with clinical problems, and even worsen them. For example, poverty might provoke and worsen experiences of worthlessness. Such depressive ideation might be a point of engagement in clinical diagnosis, while poverty is not.

What is interesting about the criteria Cooper (2005) puts forward is that they are formal, and do not focus on specific contents. This is important if one wants to avoid societal moral standards ("a good child is quiet," "a good employee is focused," etc.) determining decisions as to whether an individual's functioning is abnormal or pathological. In his three key books from the early twentieth century—*The Interpretation of Dreams* (1900), *The Psychopathology of Everyday Life* (1901), and *The Jokes and their Relation to the Unconscious* (1905)—Freud addressed the naïvety of a content-oriented approach to psychopathology, pointing out that there is no such thing as abnormal mental contents. Take a random individual's dreams and fantasies, add to these the topics she jokes about and the numerous odd events happening to her during the day; there you have a cocktail of thoughts and tendencies that do not fit with social conventions. No one is free from intentions that are mad, bad, or sad. That is why, from a Lacanian point of view, subjectivity is seen as divided in nature: often, mental representations are conflictual and rarely make up a smooth whole. In this respect, diagnostic practices that aim to distinguish between normal and abnormal thoughts and behaviors based only on their contents are naïve. A far more interesting diagnostic perspective concerns the way in which someone deals with the strange elements that manifest in one's own mental life.

Psychopathology Versus Abnormality

In his writings on the topic of diagnosis, the French philosopher and physician Georges Canguilhem (1966) makes an interesting distinction between *psychopathology* and *abnormality*, thus paving the way for the studies of Michel Foucault on the themes of psychiatric power and biopolitics. In Canguilhem's view, decision-making about normality and abnormality is generally based on two factors. First, one starts from the observation of variability in the way human beings function: individuals present with a range of behaviors just as their mental life is characterized by a diversity of beliefs and experiences, of which some are more prevalent than others. Then, a judgment is made about normality versus abnormality, which is based on a norm or standard against which behaviors are evaluated and considered as deviant or not. At this level, two possibilities open up: a judgment is made based on psychosocial criteria or statistical norms.

If the judgment is based on psychosocial criteria, it is the extent to which the individual's functioning fits his environment that is assessed. Following this logic, behavior is "normal" if nobody is particularly concerned about it, or if it doesn't cause others inconvenience. Such a line of reasoning might seem plausible, but it is based on the idea that individuals must adapt to their context: "To define abnormality in terms of social maladaptation is more or less to accept the idea that the individual must subscribe to the fact of such a society, hence must accommodate himself to it as to a reality which is at the same time a good" (Canguilhem 1966, p. 283). As social conventions change over time, identical modes of human functioning will be judged differently. The case of homosexuality illustrates this well: in the early twentieth century homosexuality was mainly seen as a moral aberration; and in the works of early sexologists homosexuality was classified as a perversion. This gave rise to the medicalized idea of homosexuality as a mental disorder. However, following societal protest in the 1970s, homosexuality was gradually accepted as a sexual orientation, alongside heterosexuality.

Applied to the DSM-5 it can be concluded that some disorders, especially those diagnosed in children, are strongly based on judgment in lieu of norms that are imposed onto the individual. For example, the criteria for diagnosing ADHD exclusively build on third-party opinions about a child, and use common sense ideas about desired behaviors in specific contexts (e.g., school) as the standard against which behaviors are evaluated. ADHD diagnostic criteria include characteristics like "Often does not seem to listen when spoken to directly (e.g., mind seems elsewhere, even in the absence of any obvious distraction)," or "Often has difficulty waiting his or her turn (e.g., while waiting in line)" (DSM-5, pp. 59–60). In the DSM-5, and other relevant literature, these diagnostic criteria are rarely discussed, leaving all interpretation as to (a) what is meant by the term "often," and (b) why specific behaviors are deemed problematic, down to the judging diagnostician. Thus, it is the professional's personal *opinions* that function as the norm against which an individual is evaluated. In other words, because stringent scientific standards for making such evaluations simply do not exist, the *belief system* of the diagnostician and his colleagues determine the standard. This can provoke overdiagnosis (Frances 2013), especially if particular professionals are inclined to problematize particular behaviors, like the teacher in my previous example. Conversely, it might equally give rise to underdiagnosis: a most tolerant diagnostician, who embraces the ideal human diversity, or who believes that nowadays far too many people are diagnosed, might qualify many behaviors and complaints as "normal," thus rendering these as not amenable for diagnosis. In both cases it is the diagnostician's opinion and not the diagnosed's distress that makes up the point of departure.

Within this view, normality comes down to an individual's adherence to normative standards of functioning, which are time- and (sub-)culture-dependent. Paul Verhaeghe (2004) notes that already in the earliest Western essays on psychology, such normative reasoning can be found. The 1590 essay by philosopher Rudolph Goclenius entitled "Psychologia: hoc est, De hominis perfectione, animo et in primis ortu hujus, commentationes ac disputationes quorundam theologorum & philosophorum nostrae aetatis" illustrates this: psychology is concerned with the perfecting of human functioning. Such a perfecting attitude seems to pervade contemporary psychological evaluation of human functioning as well. Westerners see themselves as the managers of their own life and of the life of others, and the main project they are concerned with is the manufacturing of life in terms of criteria that make one socially successful (Verhaeghe 2014). The aspiration of social success implies that norms and values held by the group dictate to the individual how he should behave. Hence Canguilhem's focus on social adaptation as one angle through which abnormality is defined.

The other option Canguilhem (1966) refers to for evaluating the normality or abnormality of human mental functioning are statistical norms.

Canguilhem indicates that such a statistically based judgment is rooted in the work of the Belgian mathematician Adolphe Quetelet (1796–1874), who aimed to study human functioning through a new discipline he coined "social physics." His underlying proposition was that social scientists should investigate and map the variability of human characteristics, ranging from physical qualities to aspects of psychological and behavioral functioning. Quetelet focused on recording how people generally function, thus giving rise to a mode of thinking in which normality is considered in terms of the *statistical normal distribution*, that is, in terms of the bell curve. In this line of reasoning normality implies a mode of functioning that closely adheres to the mean or median in statistical distribution. Abnormality, in its turn, implies a mode of functioning that strongly deviates from the average: individuals with an extreme score in terms of the normal distribution are rare or abnormal cases. Usually, the 2–10% of people deviating most strongly from the statistical norm are seen as abnormal.

Remarkably, common interpretation of statistical normal distribution frequently obtains a moral quality, meaning that significant deviation from the statistical norm is seen as indicative of deviation from normality in the moral sense of the word: significant deviation from the mean or median is evaluated as "bad" in nature. At this point moral and statistical evaluation merge: instead of using plain categorical moral criteria (e.g., "restlessness and agitation are problematic/bad"), an individual's functioning is evaluated more subtly from a dimensional perspective. This implies that traits and characteristics are still treated as morally sensitive in nature (e.g., "restlessness and agitation could be problematic/bad"), but only get sanctioned if endorsed by significant deviance from the statistical norm (e.g., "restlessness and agitation in an individual are problematic/bad if these traits are most pronounced compared to others from the same population"). Yet, statistical deviance does not imply that the extreme characteristics an individual might have are also problematic. Statistical distribution might just bear witness to variety in groups, and to variability between individuals. Variety and variability are not intrinsically good or bad, although in specific contexts extreme manifestations of certain traits might pose difficulties in interactions with others. For example, restlessness might be problematic in the kind of school environment that stresses ex cathedra instruction by the teacher, which forces the student into a receptive passive position that some have difficulty with. Thus considered, if restlessness poses problems it tells us just as much about the individual student's habits and inclinations as it does about the school context that frowns upon such behavior.

Psychological testing practices might play an important role in such a statistically based evaluation of abnormality. Often, test responses are not seen as codified responses to standardized triggers, which might further be explored through interview and observation, but are merely quantified with the aim of making comparisons with reference groups: an individual's score is compared to cut-off values that are listed in norm tables. Such tables are composed of scores obtained by administering the same test in large populations (clinical and/or non-clinical). To evaluate the individual's test score, professionals often only compare it to the distribution of scores in the general population, and along this way determine whether it deviates from the norm or not. According to Nikolas Rose (1999, p. 7) psychological tests thus provide "a mechanism for rendering subjectivity into thought as a calculable force." In his view psychological assessment and evaluation practices provide a technology, through which contemporary man inspects and perfects himself, and likewise scrutinizes and manages others. Through the lens of psychological testing, we began to think of ourselves as manageable machinery. Assessment instruments map individual differences, appraise them in terms of statistical or other social norms, and engender "techniques for the disciplining of human difference" (Rose 1999, p. 19). As the latter step is made, the group with its particular statistical distribution of scores tends to function as the moral norm against which the individual is evaluated.

As he shifts the focus from abnormality, which is appraised based on either psychosocial criteria or statistical norms, Canguilhem (1966) argues that in the diagnosis of *pathology*, the *subjective experience of human suffering* is the hallmark. Indeed, for diagnosing pathology, one cannot start from societal or statistical norms. "Pathological implies *pathos*, the direct and concrete feeling of suffering and impotence, the feeling of life gone wrong" (Canguilhem 1966, p. 137). Such a diagnosis does not build on the opinions of experts, but on *patients'* appraisal of their own distress, which tallies with Cooper's (2005) second criterion for the diagnosis of disease, which says that a condition can only be diagnosed if an individual is agonized and unhappy because of her own mental state.

Following Cooper (2005) it could be argued that in addition to the presence of pathos, which Canguilhem (1966) also stresses, psychopathology involves *moral evaluation*: pathology implies that an individual experiences aspects of her own functioning as bad. Indeed, qualifying certain experiences as good or bad implies a moral evaluation. After all, it is always in reference to standards and values that such judgments take place. Yet, while in the appraisal of normality and abnormality the opinions of others, or general tendencies in groups stand to the fore, psychopathology implies that an individual determines and evaluates her own functioning in terms of the standards and values she adheres to. Indeed, psychopathology entails an experience of falling short, which coheres with the occurrence of disruption and disturbance in the intimacy of one's own mental functioning and/or in the heart of one's relationships with others: thoughts, feelings, impulses, and actions overwhelm the individual, such that she not only feels out of control, but also believes that important norms and standards of human functioning are violated. To use a Freudian metaphor: what determines psychopathology is the acute and repetitive experience of not being the master in one's own house. For example, if an individual observes restlessness in her own functioning, which, in her opinion, undermines relational and professional functioning, restlessness makes up a relevant characteristic in terms of a diagnosis of psychopathology. This time restlessness is not problematic because others find it inappropriate, or for its exceptional intensity. What counts is the "dis-ease" it provokes in terms of how an individual fails to master what she is living through.

Obviously, psychopathology does not always involve an inward focus, with an attribution of the origin of the problem experienced to the self. For example, an individual might suffer from being persecuted by black birds that announce the arrival of Doomsday. As we focus on psychopathology, such an experience is not evaluated in terms of the incorrectness of the conviction, or in terms of the extraordinary nature of what the person is living through. What is taken into consideration is whether and how the experience baffles the individual, disrupts the ideas and norms she holds about herself and about others, and interferes with her daily functioning. In this case, an individual might feel like a defenseless victim at the mercy of a cruel other, or be perplexed with fear that she is actually going insane. What stands to the fore in both cases is the appraisal of private functioning, and the evaluation of experiences as bad/problematic in terms of her own norms and values.

However, the standards that an individual uses to evaluate her own functioning always also reflect the context the she lives in, meaning that along this way normative opinions of others have a determining effect on the appraising individual. The main difference with evaluations of normality and abnormality resides in the compulsory quality of norms and values. An individual's appraisal of psychopathology reflects her attachment to standards of functioning, but also always entails a certain amount of choice and freedom. This means that across time similar characteristics might be evaluated differently, depending on changes in the context (e.g., from unemployment to employment) and/or in her own mindset (e.g., a strong concern vs. relaxed attitude about the opinions of her parents).

What Is Pathos?

While Canguilhem's (1966) work stresses the importance of pathos in clinical diagnosis, he never fully operationalizes this concept. Indeed, Canguilhem is not focused on psychopathology and deals with the question of pathology in a generic way. Yet, in order to make pathos operational, which is crucial from a clinical point of view, the work of French philosopher Paul Ricoeur, who combined phenomenology and hermeneutics, is noteworthy. In 1992 Ricoeur presented a paper entitled *La souffrance n'est pas la douleur—Suffering is not the same as pain*, which provides a framework on how suffering and distress are expressed. While Ricoeur explicitly indicates that his analysis is not based on clinical practice, his reflections may well be applied to psychiatric problems (see also Vanheule and Devisch 2014).

The first distinction Ricoeur makes concerns the difference between somatic pain and mental suffering. What both have in common is that they are affective experiences. Yet, whereas pain manifests as distress in the body, suffering is a mental experience that is related to the language-based reflections we make about ourselves and about others. Both are distressing events we all live through at one time or another. For example, when we lose a longed-for job, or when a loved one dies we suffer, which gives rise to mourning. In such a context, Freud (1917) argues that mourning consumes the one who is left behind and is faced with the work of revising her representations of reality: raw sorrow ravages the soul. If applied to psychiatric diagnosis it could be argued that in a number of psychiatric conditions, like in severe panic, somatization, and hypochondria, pain and mental suffering are not clearly separated. Yet, what Ricoeur's analysis suggests is that logically speaking, they can be discerned, while experientially pain and suffering might present as enmeshed phenomena. Frequently, patients experience psychic pain as more severe and less tolerable than somatic pain (Yager 2015).

Ricoeur stresses that a key characteristic of suffering qua mental experience is that it cannot be measured in a standardized way. Whereas a thermometer can assist us in discerning fever in the body and medical imaging can allow us to observe brain damage, pathos cannot be measured via precise technical devices. Ricoeur indicates that we must "read" people's distress by paying attention to "signs of suffering." Suffering is neither self-evident nor open to empirical observation: It can only be discerned when people express what they live through, whether through words, somatic phenomena, or behavior, indicating a certain despair that overwhelms them.

It could be argued that since Ricoeur, instruments to assess mental suffering have been developed (Yager 2015). Indeed, a number of self-report questionnaires to assess psychic pain, like the Mental Pain Scale (Orbach et al. 2003), have been created. Next to such direct measures of mental suffering, instruments that assess disability due to mental health problems, like the Whodas 2.0 (World Health Organization 2010) which offers self-administered, proxy-administered an interviewer-administered versions, could also be seen as indicators for mental suffering. However, these instruments are all questionnaires, that don't immediately tap into the experience of suffering, but aim to grasp expressions of mental suffering in fixed formats. Such instruments provide a standardized language through which people can express themselves, assuming that in making the move from private experience to shared communication (through set

```
                    Self
                     ▲
                     |
Languishing  ◄───────┼───────►  Acting
                     |
                     ▼
                   Other
```

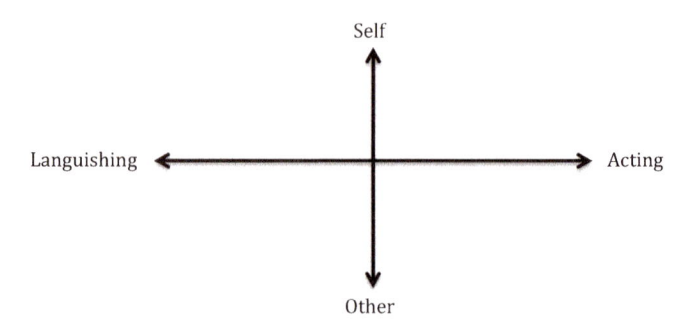

Fig. 4.1 Two orthogonal axes on which Ricoeur situates mental suffering

response categories) the essence of their experience is captured.[1] Clinically speaking, such instruments are limited in that they don't allow a complaint to be expressed in terms of the patient's own discursive repertoire, meaning that they make the patient dependent on the discourse of the professional. As already discussed in Chap. 2, such a practice exposes the patient to power dynamics in which the professional dominates.

In his conceptual model, Ricoeur discerns two orthogonal axes on which he situates mental suffering, which we represent in Fig. 4.1. There we see that pathos can be thought of in terms of the relationship between *self* and *other*, and in terms of a continuum between *languishing* (*pâtir*) and *acting* (*agir*).

In terms of the *self-other* relationship, Ricoeur suggests that suffering consists of withdrawing from the bond with the other. Those who suffer detach from others, and thus feel isolated and personally overwhelmed by the misery they endure. Such isolation renders the individual ensnared by an intolerable experience: life starts being a living hell; "the world no longer comes across as liveable, but as emptied" (Ricoeur 1992, p. 17).

---

[1] Studies using these instruments indicate that qua symptom mental suffering is indeed distinguishable from other psychiatric symptoms. Psychic pain, or psychache, is an indicator for the severity of a psychopathological condition, and of suicidality, and patients often experience it as much harder to tolerate than somatic pain, to which it is often linked. Yager (2015, p. 941) hypothetically suggests: "psychic pain might be experienced as gut-wrenching, teeth-gnashing anguish that often seems embedded in noxious somatic sensations, which, one might speculate, result from the fact that the neural networks serving these pain functions highly overlap."

In some clinical contexts withdrawal alternates with attempts to affiliate. In that case, the patient still addresses others in an attempt to express her struggle to cope. In other patients, by contrast, trust in the support of others is minimal. Indeed, in clinical problems like acute psychosis with delusions of reference or in cases of chronic abuse, disconnection from others is often more radical: the belief that the other could possibly understand what one is living through is simply missing. Sometimes the other is seen as the aggressor from which nothing positive can come, which only heightens the experience of psychological isolation and, thus, intensifies psychological suffering.

In terms of the dimension between *languishing* and *acting*, Ricoeur argues that pathos implies an experience of impossibility at the level of performing an act that could transform one's self-experience. He situates this impossibility at four levels.

First, suffering is often marked by *impossibility at the level of speech*. This is characterized by something of a fracture between two tendencies: while the patient would like to speak about what she lives through, she cannot find the right words or the courage to speak, thus ending up in silence. When speech fails in a radical way, mental suffering finds expression in crude and rudimentary (non-verbal) manifestations, like inconsolable weeping, restlessness, agonized crying, or self-harm. Here the individual is overwhelmed by destructive inner tension, which from a Lacanian point of view comes down to a *jouissance* she cannot articulate. If speech is possible, this kind of distress can prompt a minimal appeal for "help" or can be expressed in verbal complaints ("I can't live like this anymore"). Such expressions open up the possibility of a dialog and can be the impetus for integrating the painful experience into a broader narrative. Dialogical interventions, which are often successful for patients in severe distress (e.g., Seikkula et al. 2006), build on the continued effort of trying to integrate baffling experiences of distress in conversations that aim at getting hold of distress-provoking circumstances.

Second, Ricoeur situates the impossibility of acting at the level of *general passivity* and a basic inability to take action. Often, she who suffers would like to do something, but believes that nothing can be done, thus giving rise to a position in which one has to endure one's state of agony. Indeed, often patients suffering from mental pain have the feeling that they are caught in a vicious cycle, where nothing can alleviate their experience. This might drive the individual to despair. When an individual has the impression that she can link concrete actions as potential solutions to her experiences, a shift along this dimension (i.e., toward taking action) occurs. For example, a man who indicates that dark thoughts disappear for a while when playing the piano, or a mother who indicates that her baby stops crying when she lets him rest on her body, bears witness to basic steps toward overcoming the position of passivity with respect to an otherwise overwhelming psychological experience.

The third point in which Ricoeur situates the impossibility of performing an act is in *failing narration*. In line with many other scholars (e.g., Bruner 1990; Damasio 2010) Ricoeur (1992, p. 21) believes that the way in which we experience ourselves and the world is largely narratively based: "a life is nothing but the story of this life, and a quest of narration. Understanding oneself comes down to being capable of telling stories about oneself that are both intelligible and acceptable." The underlying idea is that our experiences are not inherently organized; such organization is inaugurated precisely by speaking about oneself and about the world. In the experience of pathos, such organization is missing: "suffering is expressed as a rupture in the narrative thread" (Ricoeur 1992, p. 22). Indeed, often patients who suffer can hardly speak about the things happening to them. Speaking might be too threatening, too painful or experienced as an impossible or shameful endeavor. This confronts the patient with a chaotic gap in the midst of self-experience, which some psychiatric patients fail to overcome, resulting in a continuous struggle (O'Loughlin et al. 2014). Moreover, if this narrative thread is broken, the experience of time becomes seriously altered: the future and the past lose sense, and what one is left with is the burden of the actual moment. This viewpoint tallies with Eric Cassell's (2004) idea of suffering. He stresses that events that threaten the intactness of a person, and consequently imply a perceived impending destruction or dissolution, result in suffering.

The fourth, and final, point Ricoeur refers to is the *impossibility of valuing* oneself. People only make the step toward performing an act if they think of themselves as agents that are capable of making accurate judgments. In Ricoeur's view, suffering individuals break down at this level. They no longer know if they can really trust their own opinions and appreciations of what goes on in their life, and are unsure about what they want and what they don't want. At the level of self-experience, this might lead to the conclusion of being stuck in a dead-end situation ("I'm incapable of overcoming this"), followed by inevitable feelings of guilt and shame concerning their sense of impotence in overcoming their despair. In some patients, negative self-appraisal can obtain an interpersonal quality as well, giving rise to the sense that others cannot be trusted: others cannot possibly comprehend what they are living through; they have malignant intentions in relation to which one is nothing but an object.

Next to these four aspects of impossibility in performing an act that could transform one's self-experience, Ricoeur indicates that pathos not only comes down to an experience of impossibility, but also coheres with a sense of being overwhelmed by excess. A person who suffers is devastated by a surplus of affective stimuli that cannot be contained by means of words and actions. Inner tension, which, in clinical contexts, is frequently felt through bodily sensations that do not spontaneously resolve, hence suffering individuals' tendencies to act upon the body (e.g., through self-harm or substance abuse), or to externalize overwhelming strain (e.g., through aggressive acts).

Finally, suffering usually gives rise to a plethora of questions that simply cannot be answered in straightforward ways; answers are incessantly sought nevertheless: "Indeed, questioning is related to plaints: Until when? Why me? Why my child?" (Ricoeur 1992, p. 30). Suffering not only has a perplexing effect, it provokes a perpetual search for sense and reason concerning the *why and wherefore* of one's experience.

Considered from Lacan's theory, suffering not only confronts the human being with a senseless element of *jouissance*, which is felt as a strain, but also confronts her with the question of her own existence. As we suffer, we face an unintelligible component that disturbs our common inner world. It actualizes a "something-else" or an "Other-thing" that concerns us, yet, cognizing efforts fail to get hold of such a disturbing experience. In terms of Lacanian terminology, suffering presents us with a so-called *extimate* element: a strange component in the interiority of our intimate experience. Lacan (1959, p. 459) suggests that given human self-reflexivity, which coheres with our use of signifiers, such an experience confronts us with a basic question: "Who am I?" Suffering challenges what, and how we habitually think of ourselves and of others, which gives rise to self-directed epistemic questions ("What/who am I?") and to questions concerning the opinions and intentions of others in relation to us ("What does he/she want?")." Thus considered, mental suffering entails much more than the experience of debilitating symptoms. It coheres with a painful intimate interrogation, which, quite characteristically, crystalizes around the identity-related topics humans usually struggle with, like gender identity, parenthood, or the meaning of life. From a Lacanian point of view such a link between mental suffering and identity-related questions are not surprising. Lacanian theory presumes that confrontations with identity-related issues might give rise to inner conflict, or have a maddening traumatic impact, which makes up the breeding ground for symptoms and suffering.

A Plea for Studying the Quality and Circumstances of Mental Suffering

What is interesting about the above analyses of mental suffering is that they urge us to study the *quality* of mental suffering: not only should we examine whether prospective patients have symptoms, above all we have to get hold of their impact on a person's functioning. Indeed, diagnosis should not be especially or exclusively concerned with grasping the syndrome a person is afflicted by, but above all with getting in touch with the sick person (Cassell 2004). Symptoms have to be situated in the context of people's life. They are indicators of crisis, and need to be studied in terms of how one relates to others, as well as to challenges one is confronted with.

In line with Canguilhem, we had better not buy into the idea that distress should be considered as a quantity that can be measured. Pathos cannot be grasped on a measurement scale, but should be studied in terms how people make sense of themselves, and act in relation to others.

As Cassell (2004, p. 42) succinctly writes: "the only way to learn whether suffering is present is to ask the sufferer." Such inquiry can be challenging, especially if one aims to avoid merely subjecting the patient to the discursively based regime of the professional. After all, in its most extreme form, pathos is expressed via withdrawal from the other, accompanied by non-verbal expressions of discontent, which is by no means immediately related to speech. Catatonia, where the patient remains immobile, apathetic, and barely able to communicate, is illustrative of this.

Following Ricoeur's two axes, pathos could be thought of as an expressive phenomenon that must be read and described. No doubt, such a reading of pathos is a person-oriented endeavor. At a clinical level, pathos should be carefully studied in each individual case concerning what the patient lives through and how they express distress. For instance, an inconsolable six-month-old baby expresses pathos differently than a toddler who simply cannot sit still. Similarly, in an adult who repeatedly and anxiously consults his physician, pathos is expressed in a manner that is quite distinct from the recluse who believes that others are perpetually mocking him. As a consequence, diagnosticians must above all *describe* and *document* as specifically as possible how an individual expresses the particularity of what the DSM-5 has rather vacantly termed "distress." Professionals should have an eye, and an ear, for how the patient's symptoms generate isolation from others. Likewise, it should be taken into account that suffering is often expressed through impasses: the inability to speak, take action, narrate, and value oneself.

In terms of practical clinical reality, this viewpoint implies that mapping suffering and distress entails a lot more than administering self-report questionnaires or completing checklist scores. Following Ricoeur's analysis, in the attempt to quantify mental suffering many of its qualities get lost: its embedment in a life, and in specific living conditions, cannot be grasped in numbers. This does not imply that all standardized measurement scales have little use. Questionnaires may occupy a meaningful role in diagnostic practice. Questionnaire scores might provide useful indications that can alert clinicians to the *presence* of mental suffering in an individual, yet an appraisal of the person's experience of pathos requires a narratively based qualitative approach.

Practically speaking, this implies that clinicians' ideas about patients' distress should be embedded in *case formulations* or *case constructions*. Case formulations are narratives in which clinicians single out essential information about a case and integrate their findings in a tentative explanatory structure (Sturmey 2009). Characteristically, case formulations discuss core symptoms and key clinical characteristics in a patient's functioning, with the aim of getting hold of structural patterns and singular incidents that elucidate why an individual functions the way she does. Fine-grained descriptions of how mental suffering manifests, and of the circumstances in which it takes shape, are crucial to such a construction. Indeed, key to case formulations is that they don't only have a descriptive aim. Rather than making a tailor-made list of the problems a patient suffers from, case constructions should aim at getting hold of *conditions, constellations, and dynamics* that have a *positive or negative impact* on a person's functioning. What thus stands to the fore is the contextual embedment relative to life events, life history, living conditions, and relational functioning.

When clinicians discuss patients, their focus is often mainly directed toward factors that undermine mental consistency, that is, to what goes wrong in patients' life. Recent debates on mental health and mental illness increasingly pay attention to factors that make up strengths and stabilizing factors in persons' functioning (e.g., Manwell et al. 2015). Such a focus not only broadens the scope, but might also help individuals to function more independently from power regimes in psychiatry. In terms of Lacan's later theoretical elaborations, which strongly builds on mathematical knot theory, this implies that attention should not be exclusively directed toward issues that untie the knot of mental functioning, but also explicitly to factors that help find consistency, and keep the disorienting Real at bay. An interesting example Lacan (1975–1976) discussed in this context is the writer James Joyce. In Joyce's functioning strange peculiarities can be found, like an odd relation to language, to his body, to fame, and to his relatives. Lacan does not discuss these oddities in terms of the mental condition Joyce might have suffered from, but examines what it was that provided the writer with satisfactory mental stability, and prevented him from ending up in madness. Despite the traits that might make Joyce look abnormal, Lacan focuses on aspects in Joyce's functioning that provided him with stability, and prevented him from going mad.

His art of writing and the cult that he created around himself as a writer were crucial in this context. Indeed, in the same vein, case constructions should not only focus on dynamics that give rise to symptoms and suffering, but equally pay attention to factors that protect a person from ending up in suffering.

Which position does the DSM take in this debate? With respect to case formulations the answer is straightforward. While the manual recognizes the value of case construction, it does not qualify it as the heart of diagnostic activity, which is reflected in its focus on checklists. The DSM-5 (p. 19) devotes two paragraphs to the idea that diagnostic conclusions should indeed be embedded in clinical case formulations, but does not provide details on the characteristics of a good clinical case formulation, and above all seems to communicate that what really matters is diagnostic classification.

DSM-5: A Matter of Disorders

In the previous sections we made a contrast between the concepts "psychopathology" and "abnormality," assuming that diagnosis should especially focus on psychopathology, that is, on the difficulties a person experiences in aspects of her own functioning, focusing on how she suffers. Thus considered diagnosis is concerned with the way in which one relates to oneself and to others, and with the question as to whether pathos enters into this experience. If the focus remains only on abnormality, by contrast, external norms and opinions of others stand to the fore. Characteristically, individuals that cause hindrance in relation to others, and people whose psychosocial functioning deviates quite strongly from the average, are candidates for such an abnormality diagnosis. A further question we can ask is which position the DSM takes in this discussion.

In the introductory pages of DSM-5 (p. 20) the following definition of mental disorder can be found:

> A mental disorder is a syndrome characterized by clinically significant disturbance in an individual's cognition, emotion regulation, or behavior that reflects a dysfunction in the psychological, biological, or developmental

processes underlying mental functioning. Mental disorders are usually associated with significant distress or disability in social, occupational, or other important activities. An expectable or culturally approved response to a common stressor or loss, such as the death of a loved one, is not a mental disorder. Socially deviant behavior (e.g., political, religious, or sexual) and conflicts that are primarily between the individual and society are not mental disorders unless the deviance or conflict results from a dysfunction in the individual, as described above.

This definition indicates that, above all, mental disorders are conceptualized as typical sets of symptoms and clinically observable signs that make up a syndromic whole. It is presumed that these syndromes are indicative of an "underlying dysfunction" in the psychological, biological, or developmental sphere. As discussed in the previous chapters, such a focus on underlying dysfunction reflects a decontextualized and reifying view, which neglects the constructed nature of mental symptoms.

However, above all the idea of *dysfunction*, which is a concept the DSM does not explain any further, seems to assume that we have a clear idea on what effective and efficient psychological, biological, or developmental functioning implies. Such a line of reasoning strongly rests on the assumption that our mental apparatus functions along the lines of a biological and evolutionarily designed blueprint, which is not adequately working in case of mental disorder. The main problem is that scientists actually don't know how "functional" mental activity would be organized, and as a result all evaluations of dysfunction rest on value-laden assessments. For example, an individual might develop depressive symptoms in a job context where harsh interactions and bullying make up daily reality. What would be characteristic of a biologically and evolutionary functional reaction to a bullying boss? Some people deal with such a situation in silence, focusing on their work-related activities as much as possible, thus aiming to keep painful interactions at a distance. Others lose all interest in their job, and become consumed with anger and a desire to strike back. Which reaction is functional and which one dysfunctional? The DSM cannot resolve this dilemma, and also does not frame it in terms of context and subjective experience, but switches to normative decision-making focusing on the normality and abnormality of specific behaviors. According to Jerome Wakefield, it sanctions behaviors in terms of how unusual they are in the general population. Along this way the manual "replaces the dysfunction requirement with the requirement that the condition cannot be a statistically expectable response to the environment" (Wakefield 1992, p. 233). Dysfunction cannot be adequately defined; therefore, the DSM takes an a priori focus on behavioral traits, thus sanctioning extreme modes of behavior and experience. In his analysis Wakefield builds quite strongly on the idea that it is particularly the statistically extreme behaviors that have entered the DSM checklists. This may in part be true, but one can also see that the criteria just as much reflect stark moral judgments on behaviors that others do not tolerate. The ADHD criteria illustrate this well.

In his work on the concept of mental disorder Jerome Wakefield (1992, 2010), who actually criticizes the DSM definition, maintains a focus on dysfunction, suggesting that we should think of mental disorders as "harmful dysfunctions." In his view, dysfunction involves "a failure of some mental mechanism to perform one of its natural or biological functions, as judged by evolutionary biological design," while harmfulness implies a normative judgment: "The value or 'harm' component refers to negative or undesirable or harmful conditions as judged by social values" (Wakefield 2010, p. 343). What is problematic about this definition is that it again builds on the idea of evolutionarily designed mental functions which might be hampered or not, while the exact methods and norms to assess irregularities in individuals' mental functioning do not exist (see also Cooper 2005). Interestingly, Wakefield (2010) also stresses the value-laden dimension of diagnosis: symptoms are embedded in contexts, and have a moral meaning that coheres with the context and the individual. Along this way, he warns us against a normative approach to dysfunction that only starts from opinions of others and statistical information about human functioning, thus making a plea for us to take into account the diagnosed person's perspective in diagnostic evaluations. The DSM, by contrast, does not specify the necessity to build on the subjective experience of the individual who is diagnosed. As a result, deviance from the statistical mean, and opinions of others concerning the unacceptability of someone's behavior, tend to be central to the evaluation of dysfunction.

Indeed, while the definition subsequently specifies that "usually" mental disorders are associated with "significant distress," it does not assume that the symptom and mental suffering are inherently connected. This ambiguity implies that diagnoses might be given while the diagnosed individual does not suffer from what she lives through. A further major ambiguity can be found in the last sentence of the definition, which says that socially deviant behaviors and conflicts are not indicative of mental disorder, unless the deviance or conflict results from a dysfunction. Given the absence of a straightforward definition of dysfunction, and the observation that in practice dysfunction is evaluated starting from social value criteria, this specification in the last sentence of the DSM definition actually seems to confirm that while a link with mental symptoms is needed, evaluating social nuisance is pivotal to the DSM.

Going against our emphasis on mental suffering, which could be seen as too person-focused, it might be argued that actually the DSM does well in saying that mental disorders can be linked with disability in social functioning. Such a broadening focus might indeed be relevant. Yet, again the DSM does not specify how disabilities should be conceptualized. The concept "disability" is complex, and has a long history (Mallet and Runswikc-Cole 2014). The World Health Organization currently defines it as "an umbrella term for impairments, activity limitations, and participation restrictions. Disability refers to the negative aspects of the interaction between individuals with a health condition (such as cerebral palsy, Down syndrome, depression) and personal and environmental factors (such as negative attitudes, inaccessible transportation and public buildings, and limited social supports)" (WHO 2011b, p. 7). What is important about this definition is that disability is not an individual problem, but a contextual and interactional phenomenon: "disability results from the interaction between persons with impairments and attitudinal and environmental barriers that hinder their full and effective participation in society on an equal basis with others" (WHO 2011a, p. 4). In line with this definition, many mental health problems imply significant disability, which, for example, can be observed in a reduced capacity to participate in mainstream jobs and schools. Often, people with symptoms are hampered by prejudice because of unusual aspects in their modes of functioning. Prejudice and rejection obstruct social interaction. The WHO definition implies that disability is an outcome of the *interaction* between an individual and a context, which both have peculiarities. Indeed, disability is not simply a personal trait that can be attributed to an individual, but is just as much an expression of how the context around an individual is organized, and how contextual mechanisms of exclusion hamper the individual. Thus considered, the WHO disability diagnosis goes hand in hand with empowerment-oriented thinking. Given the fact that social environments are shaped by social values, this viewpoint implies that, in part, disability is caused by the context. Disability holds up a mirror to the context, and points to expectations and elements of prejudice, through which an individual is judged, just as it reflects idiosyncrasies in an individual's functioning. By leaving disability undefined, and not embracing such an interactional perspective, the DSM, by contrast, might well entail an individualizing focus, in which disability is seen as an outcome of personal dysfunction. Moreover, it is unclear whose perspective is taken as a reference in the DSM assessment of disability. Clearly, the WHO definition implies that the position of the individual who experiences disability stands to the fore. Conversely, DSM-oriented diagnosis might well imply that opinions of others, like parents' and teachers' beliefs about a child, prevail. The DSM definition of mental disorder not only leaves disability undefined, but also juxtaposes it with mental distress. This implies that diagnoses might be given if only a disability is experienced, and no distress. This is a problem given the fact that the DSM does not specify that disability needs to be assessed in terms of participation restrictions.

Indeed, in terms of our discussion of psychopathology and abnormality the DSM account of mental disorder is ambiguous. On the one hand it suggests that distress and disability should be taken into account, but on the other hand, doing so is not a necessary condition, which shows that pathos is not its real focus. Actually, above all, the DSM builds on an assessment of abnormality. To a large extent, the disorder checklists itemize extreme or unusual behaviors and experiences that were formulated by key opinion leaders, and the frequency and intensity with which such traits manifest in an individual determine the diagnosis.

Historically speaking, the specification of distress in mental disorders first appeared in the DSM-III. The two previous versions of the manual did not contain such a specification, and left the concept of mental disorder largely undefined. A section on how mental disorders could be defined was added following heated discussions in the 1970s concerning homosexuality (Decker 2013; Kutchins and Kirk 1997). Whereas in the DSM-II homosexuality was included as a mental disorder, Robert Spitzer, the president of the DSM-III taskforce, came to the conclusion that many homosexuals did not suffer from their sexual preference, but from society's reactions to it. Fellow psychiatrists who were homosexual, as well as gay activists, convinced Spitzer that they had no mental illness. In order to avoid misdiagnosis the category of homosexuality was replaced by "ego-dystonic homosexuality" in the DSM-III. The main difference between non-problematic, ego-syntonic homosexuality and the ego-dystonic variant is that the latter provokes distress, while the former does not. In general, Spitzer concluded that the experience of distress is central to the diagnosis of mental disorders, hence its inclusion in the overall definition of mental disorder (Decker 2013; Kutchins and Kirk 1997). However, what Spitzer failed to do was include distress as a necessary condition for a diagnosis of mental disorder. Nowadays, the DSM is still ambiguous with respect to the status of mental suffering (Bolton 2013). It only says "Mental disorders are *usually* associated with significant distress or disability" (DSM-5, p. 20, our italics), which implies that it remains possible that psychiatric diagnoses are given to individuals that don't subjectively suffer from aspects of their own mental functioning: the DSM suggests that the experience of pathos is important, but what really counts is the presence of abnormalities in mental functioning.

What About Suffering: *Verstehen* or *Gardez-vous de comprendre*?

If diagnosis comes down to constructing case formulations in which symptoms are framed in the context of a person's broader functioning, such that the impairing impact of symptom and context, the logic of functioning, as well as strengths and aspects of resilience are mapped, the main question remains as to which position the clinician should take in dealing with the highly subjective material obtained about the patient's functioning. Some clinicians will stress that obtaining genuine understanding of what the patient lives through is crucial, while others clearly have reservations regarding such an attempt to understand.

According to Karl Jaspers (1912), who is a key figure in phenomenological approaches to psychiatry, building a deliberate and effortful understanding of what the patient lives through is crucial. In his approach the diagnostician should not only describe the patient's problems, but aim at understanding them, and thus at getting hold of why and how given symptoms come hand in hand with the experience of suffering. Just as Ricoeur did in his wake, Jaspers states that by using standardized measurement instruments one cannot adequately assess mental processes. To get hold of the precise nature and of the impact of mental health symptoms we have to build on people's speech, and on the opinions they have about their own experiences. In doing so a three-step trajectory needs to be explored.

In the first step, clinicians should adequately describe complaints and related experiences: "We must begin with a clear representation of what is actually going on in the patient, what he is really experiencing, how things arise in his consciousness, what are his own feelings, and so forth" (Jaspers 1912, p. 1316). Along this way an inventory of painful aspects in the patient's experience is made. Important to this phenomenological approach is that the clinician does not "translate" the patient's speech in professional discourse ("you have a depression, sir"), but explores it in terms of the patient's meaning-making activities: "the aim of phenomenological investigation is the description of the lived experience, a description of phenomena just as they present themselves or are given in experience" (Parnas and Zahavi 2000, p. 12).

Jaspers indicates that in the next step, the clinician should map the context and circumstances in which the described mental phenomena are embedded: "We have to be led, starting from the outside, to a real appreciation of a particular psychic phenomenon by looking at its genesis, the conditions for its appearance, its configurations, its context and possible concrete contents" (Jaspers 1912, p. 1316). In this second step, descriptively mapped phenomena can be contextualized, starting from the patient's perceptions and appreciations of specific symptoms.

While these first steps reflect an overall clinical attitude that connects well with the biographical tradition in nineteenth-century psychiatry (Berrios 1992), the third step Jaspers envisions is quite specific to phenomenological approaches, and consists of creating a deep empathic understanding (*Verstehen*) of what the patient lives through. The clinician should not only "know" what goes on in the patient, but also "see" the patient's perspective by actualizing it in his own mind: "Just as sense-perceptions are evoked by the demonstration of an object, so this meaningful empathic actualization will be evoked in us by the above-mentioned hints and indications, by our immediate grasp of expressive phenomena and our self-immersion in other people's self-description" (Jaspers 1912, p. 1317). By being a mirror for the other's intimate experiences, the phenomenologically working clinician aims at grasping the patient's mental symptoms and suffering. Such empathic understanding comes down to an imaginary identification: the clinician builds an image of what the other lives through, and identifies with this image, such that the other's state of being can be experienced. The French philosopher Emmanuel Lévinas (1982) even adds a step to the threefold process Jaspers describes, suggesting that understanding is not enough. In his view we should not only comprehend the patient's suffering, but also suffer ourselves with the patient, which is the only way to get hold of the patient's distress (Gantt 2000).

On a critical note it could be added that not all clinicians are equally enthusiastic about such an effort of empathic understanding. Lacan's (1955–1956) criticism is in this context illustrative. In his view deliberate empathic actualization does not necessarily result in a better appraisal of patients' difficulties, but might as well have a reverse effect. After all, a fundamental problem with it is that it takes the clinician's experience as the standard, and always starts from the clinician's ideas on what plausibly goes on in the patient, while nothing guarantees that the clinician can adequately grasp the patient's mind. For example, this is also what a study on empathic accuracy in psychology students shows (Barone et al. 2005). Researchers videotaped a therapy session, and subsequently asked the patient what she thought and felt at different moments during the session. After watching the session students also had to describe what, in their view, the patient was living through. The results indicate that while students' appraisals of emotions were sometimes similar to those the patient revealed, the patient's thoughts could not be grasped properly. Subsequent training sessions had a positive effect on both facets of empathic understanding, but the net result is that empathic accuracy remains limited.

Clearly, the effort of empathic understanding has a number of positive effects. It creates a bond between the clinician and patient, and the quality of this relationship predicts recovery (Blatt and Zuroff 2005). Through its use of imaginary identification empathic actualization often creates a link, thus engendering the belief that the patient and clinician share the same ideas. In Lacan's (1955–1956) view, such a process of attunement is inherently limited since it might well blind the clinician to inconsistencies in the patient's functioning, and make her neglect peculiarities that the patient and/or clinician prefer to set aside. Characteristic of imaginary functioning is that it tends toward building comprehensive Gestalt-like ideas, which misrecognizes incomprehensible or less imaginable elements. Empathic understanding exclusively bears witness to synthesis-oriented tendencies in mental functioning, which the clinician should temper with the aim of getting hold of symbolic and real components in the patient's functioning too (see Chap. 3). Hence Lacan's dictum (1956a, p. 394[2]): "Beware of understanding" (*Gardez-vous de comprendre*), which does not imply that the clinician should explicitly not try to understand the patient, but denotes that effortful understanding should not be thought of as the ultimate tool or the final aim in clinical work. Indeed, by addressing imaginary, symbolic, and real components in patients' suffering a more adequate case construction can be made.

Conclusion

Following the French physiologist René Leriche, Canguilhem (1966, p. 91) conceptualizes health as "life lived in the silence of the organs," and disease as "what irritates men in the normal course of their lives and

---

[2] Bruce Fink translated "Gardez-vous de comprendre" as "Don't try to understand." I believe "Beware of understanding" is better.

work, and above all, what makes them suffer." In this line of reasoning the idea of "the normal course" does not suggest that normative standards derived from the group should be applied to the individual, but to a relatively homeostatic balance in the functioning of the individual, which might be destabilized or not. In his view symptoms express global disturbance, meaning that disease requires a holistic approach that takes into account the connection between diverse aspects of an individual's functioning. Hence his idea that "the norm in pathology is above all an individual norm" (Canguilhem 1966, p. 119).

Concordant with Canguilhem's theory, *mental health* might be described as a state of functioning in which thoughts, feelings, and behaviors are self-evident to an individual, and don't make themselves heard in a self-reflective loop. *Psychopathology*, by contrast, is a mode of functioning in which thoughts, feelings, and behaviors start functioning as symptoms that actively disturb the way one wants to live, to the extent that intense suffering is produced. In line with our triangular model of symptom formation (see Chap. 3), symptoms are indicators of imbalance and conflict that take shape at the crossroad between contextual influences (individual, familial, social, and (sub-)cultural factors), physiological processes, and the act of speaking. Although language-based configuration processes determine symptoms and suffering, these, from a Lacanian point of view, also always imply a *real* component. This means that they reflect elements of inconsistency and impasse, and express an *extimate* experience of *jouissance,* which challenges the experience of identity and produces *pathos.*

Within this view, diagnosis does not come down to "syndrome labeling," but to constructing a thoughtful formulation pertaining to the conditions, constellations, and dynamics in an individual's life that make up the systemic context within which symptoms and suffering take shape. In building such case construction, clinical knowledge and theoretical models about syndromes might be helpful, but the main focus is on the abductive formulation of a framework that tentatively explains the logic within which symptoms and suffering are most plausibly embedded. Indeed, case formulation is a matter of *abductive reasoning*: starting from a specific symptom within a singular case, characteristic features of functioning are evaluated, and through addressing the question as to what might have caused the problem the most likely explanation is retained. While in psychiatric reflection, abductive reasoning often focuses on syndrome detection (Réjon Altable 2012), it might more broadly be applied to contextualizing case formulation approaches as well (Vertue and Haig 2008). What is important to such a case-construction-oriented approach to diagnosis is that while starting from what goes wrong in an individual, specific attention should also be paid to disabling factors in the relationship with the other, as well as to strengths and stability-creating factors that counter the experience of psychopathology.

Classificatory approaches to mental health problems often mainly build on a normative judgment of abnormality in terms of the statistical or societal standards the diagnostician adheres to. Along this way, the experience of psychopathology, as defined in the previous sections, is often neglected. While case formulation can just as well be used in an approach that prioritizes the diagnostician's standards, it is especially suited for taking into account a patient-based value judgment of specific thoughts, feelings, and behaviors. Case formulation might be used to articulate an ethical position that highlights the patient's position. Indeed, since diagnosis invariably implies the establishment of power regimes, great care should be taken that the patient does not receive the message that she should adapt to external norms. What should come first is the question as to how the elements of disorder the patient is living through are organized, and how these problems might be addressed in a sustainable way, such that idiosyncrasies in the patient's functioning are voiced and valued.

Other References

Barone, D. F., et al. (2005). Increasing empathic accuracy through practice and feedback in clinical interviewing course. *Journal of Social and Clinical Psychology, 24*, 156–171.

Berrios, G. E. (1992). Phenomenology, psychopathology and Jaspers: A conceptual history. *History of Psychiatry, 3*, 303–327.

Blatt, S. J., & Zuroff, D. C. (2005). Empirical evaluation of the assumptions in identifying evidence based treatments in mental health. *Clinical Psychology Review, 25*, 459–486.

Bolton, D. (2013). Overdiagnosis problems in the DSM-IV and the new DSM-5: Can they be resolved by the distress – Impairment criterion? *Canadian Journal of Psychiatry, 58,* 612–617.

Bruner, J. (1990). *Acts of meaning.* Cambridge: Harvard University Press.

Canguilhem, G. (1966). *The normal and the pathological.* Brooklyn: Zone Books.

Cassell, E. J. (2004). *The nature of suffering and the goals of medicine.* Oxford: Oxford University Press.

Cooper, R. (2005). *Classifying madness – A philosophical examination of the diagnostic and statistical manual of mental disorders.* Dordrecht: Springer.

Damasio, A. (2010). *Self comes to mind: Constructing the conscious brain.* New York: Vintage.

Decker, H. (2013). *The making of DSM-III.* New York: Oxford University Press.

Frances, A. (2013). *Saving normal – An insider's revolt against out-of-control psychiatric diagnosis, DSM-5, big pharma, and the medicalization of ordinary life.* New York: William Morrow & Harper Collins Publishers.

Freud, S. (1953 [1917]). Mourning and Melancholia. In *The standard edition of the complete psychological works for Sigmund Freud* (Vol. 14, pp. 243–258). London: Hogarth Press.

Gantt, E. E. (2000). Levinas, psychotherapy, and the ethics of suffering. *Journal of Humanistic Psychology, 40,* 9–28.

Jaspers, K. (1912). The phenomenological approach in psychopathology. *British Journal of Psychiatry, 114,* 1313–1323.

Kutchins, H., & Kirk, S. A. (1997). *Making us crazy: DSM – The psychiatric bible and the creation of mental disorders.* New York: Free Press.

Lacan, J. (1992 [1959–1960]). *The seminar, Book VII, the ethics of psychoanalysis.* London/New York: W. W. Norton.

Lacan, J. (1955–1956/1993). *The seminar 1955–1956, Book III, the psychoses.* New York/London: W.W. Norton.

Lacan, J. (2005 [1975–1976]). *Le séminaire, livre XXIII, le sinthome [The seminar, book XXIII, the sinthome].* Paris: Seuil.

Lacan, J. (2006 [1956a]). The situation of psychoanalysis and the training of psychoanalysts in 1956. In J. Lacan & J. A. Miller (Eds.), *Écrits* (pp. 384–411). New York/London: W. W. Norton.

Laroi, F. (2012). How do auditory verbal hallucinations in patients differ from those in non-patients? *Frontiers in human neuroscience, 6,* 25.

Lévinas, E. (1982). La souffrance inutile [Pointless suffering]. In E. Lévinas (Ed.), *Entre nous. Essais sur le penser-à-l'autre* (pp. 100–112). Paris: Grasset, 1993.

Manwell, L. A. et al. (2015). What is mental health? Evidence towards a new definition from a mixed methods multidisciplinary international survey. *BMJ Open, 5*, e007079. doi:10.1136/bmjopen-2014-007079Mental health.

Mallet, R., & Runswick-Cole, K. (2014). *Approaching disability: Critical issues and perspectives*. London/New York: Routledge.

O'Loughlin, M., Charles, M., Crosby, J., et al. (2014). Closing the gap: Narrating the prose of severe psychic suffering. *Psychoanalysis, Culture & Society, 19*, 98–106.

Orbach, I., Mikulincer, M., Sirota, P., et al. (2003). Mental pain: A multidimensional operationalization and definition. *Suicide and Life-Threatening Behavior, 33*, 219–230.

Parens, E., & Johnston, J. (2011). Troubled children: Diagnosing, treating and attending to context: A hastings center special report. *Hastings Center Report, 41*(2), 1–32.

Parnas, J., & Zahavi, D. (2000). The link: Philosophy-psychopathology-phenomenology. In D. Zahavi (Ed.), *Exploring the self*. Amsterdam: John Benjamins.

Réjon Altable, C. (2012). Logic structure of clinical judgment and its relation to medical and psychiatric semiology. *Psychopathology, 45*, 344–351.

Ricoeur, P. (1992/2013). La souffrance n'est pas la douleur [suffering is not the same as pain]. In C. Marin & N. Zaccaï-Reyners (Eds.), *Souffrance et douleur* (pp. 13–33). Paris: Presses Universitaires de France.

Rose, N. (1999). *Governing the soul – The shaping of the private self – Second edition*. London/New York: Free Association Books.

Seikkula, J., Aaltonen, J., Alakare, B., et al. (2006). Five-year experience of first-episode nonaffective psychosis open-dialogue approach: Treatment principles, follow-up outcomes and two case studies. *Psychotherapy Research, 16*, 214–228.

Sturmey, P. (2009). Case formulation: A review and overview of this volume. In P. Sturmey (Ed.), *Clinical case formulation: Varieties of approaches* (pp. 3–32). Oxford: Wiley-Blackwell.

Vanheule, S., & Devisch, I. (2014). Mental suffering and the DSM-5: A critical review. *The Journal of Evaluation of Clinical Practice, 20*, 975–980.

Vanheule, S., & Verhaeghe, P. (2004). Powerlessness and impossibility in special education: A qualitative study on professional burnout from a Lacanian perspective. *Human Relations, 57*, 497–519.

Verhaeghe, P. (2014). *What about me? – The struggle for identity in a market-based society*. Victoria/London: Scribe.

Vertue, F. M., & Haig, B. D. (2008). An abductive perspective on clinical reasoning and case formulation. *Journal of Clinical Psychology, 64*, 1046–1068.

Wakefield, J. C. (1992). Disorder as harmful dysfunction: A conceptual critique of DSM-II-R's definition of mental disorder. *Psychological Review, 99*, 232–247.

Wakefield, J. C. (2010). Misdiagnosing normality: Psychiatry's failure to address the problem of false positive diagnoses of mental disorder in a changing professional environment. *Journal of Mental Health, 19*, 337–351.

World Health Organization. (2010). *Measuring health and disability: Manual for WHO Disability Assessment Schedule (WHODAS 2.0)*. Geneva: World Health Organization.

World Health Organization. (2011a). *World report on disability*. Geneva: World Health Organization.

World Health Organization. (2011b). *World report on disability – Summary*. Geneva: World Health Organization.

Yager, J. (2015). Addressing patients' psychic pain. *American Journal of Psychiatry, 172*, 939–943.

5

Working with Clinical Case Formulations: Methodological Considerations

Mapping Mental Health Problems

In Chaps. 2 and 3 we focused on classificatory diagnosis, and looked critically at what kind of appraisal of mental health problems the DSM manual leads to. Reliability and validity were our core concepts. With these concepts we evaluated how solid the DSM is in assessing psychopathology in clinical practice. This brought us to the conclusion that the evidence supporting the DSM approach to mental symptoms is limited. The DSM does not enhance solid and straightforward clinical decision-making, and by decontextualizing symptoms through its mere focus on psychiatric syndromes crucial information on the meaning and function of the symptom gets lost. In Chaps. 3 and 4 we made a plea for studying the quality and the context of mental suffering. Assuming that in making a diagnosis "thorough knowledge" concerning an individual's symptoms, disability, and suffering needs to be collected, we suggested that case formulations provide us with a useful format. In case formulations symptoms are framed within the context of a person's broader functioning, such that the damaging impact of symptom and context, the logic of functioning, as well as strengths and aspects of resilience are mapped.

This chapter returns to the concepts of reliability and validity, examining how they apply to case formulations.

It is generally accepted that a measurement instrument is *reliable* if it allows us to draw conclusions in a consistent way. Studies show that the reliability of psychiatric decision-making is far from obvious. This applies both to the recent versions of the DSM and to older diagnostic systems. Many idiosyncratic factors seem to have a great impact, such that in a large number of cases professionals assess the same patient differently to their colleagues. Some will be annoyed when reading that idiosyncratic factors play such an important role in psychiatric diagnosis. Nevertheless, we argue that these factors are not arbitrary and that professionals must do everything in their power to assess patients' symptoms and suffering as accurately as possible. However, if we accept the proposal of Marková and Berrios (2009), or our Triangular Model of Symptom Formation, which suggest that psychological symptoms are not natural objects that we can observe, but constructed phenomena, we cannot but bring subjectivity into account. Not only are patients' experiences of symptoms constructed in an interplay between physical, psychological, social, and cultural factors, but professionals also grant meaning to the actions and words of the patient. Herewith they too are influenced by many factors, such as their socio-cultural background, professional training, and life experiences (Did you ever hear voices? Have you ever lost a friend through suicide?).

Validity relates to the correctness of measurements. A measuring instrument is valid if it really assesses what one wishes to know. In Chap. 3 we suggested that forms of psychopathology come to be through a subjective construction process. We emphasized that psychological configuration processes and context factors play an important role in the creation of psychological symptoms. Whoever experiences symptoms not only endures them passively, but also experiences them qua self-reflexive transcendental subject. The DSM does not bring these configuration processes and the self-reflexive relationship of people to their symptoms into account, and therefore does not provide a valid appreciation of psychopathology. Moreover, the DSM-5 starts from the idea that mental disorders are biologically founded. Meanwhile research largely contradicts this and points to a complex interplay between biological, social, and psychological factors, which implies that in accordance with its own biological aspirations, the validity of the DSM-5 leaves much to be desired.

That there are major issues concerning the clinical value and the scientific quality of the DSM will have become clear. It is therefore not wise to organize scientific research, clinical work, or the organization of mental health care too strongly on the basis of this psychiatric manual.

A simple alternative to the DSM, however, does not exist. Switching to a different classification system cannot solve crucial problems with this form of diagnosis. In accordance with our contextualizing ideas about psychological symptoms, diagnosis should not primarily focus on the detection of disorders, but on a clarification of the *role and function of a symptom* within someone's functioning. Diagnosis in the field of mental health should be function-oriented rather than disorder-oriented. In this chapter I further discuss what function-oriented diagnosis by means of case formulations implies, and discuss how the validity and the reliability of this narrative form of diagnosis can be optimized. Just as my criticism of the DSM in Chaps. 2 and 3 is especially methodological in nature, I focus my discussion of function-oriented diagnosis especially on methodological aspects of clinical case formulation. A methodological framework for the work with case formulations is essential to give shape to a theory-based function-oriented appraisal of mental symptoms, disability, and suffering.

Function-Oriented Diagnosis

In order to introduce function-oriented diagnosis I return to Freud, in whose work a subtle but important shift in the use of the concept "diagnosis" stands out. Where he uses the term "diagnosis" initially in the classic medical meaning to refer to a set of disease symptoms that together constitute a disease entity such as hysteria, we notice from his case study on Dora (Freud 1905b) that he also uses the term in a different way. This happens very concretely when he writes about Dora's aphony—suddenly she is no longer able to speak. Freud notes that the symptom is related to the absence of her beloved, which brings him to the next question: "Am I now going on to assert that in every instance in which there are periodical attacks of aphonia we are to diagnose the existence of a loved person who is at times away from the patient?" (Freud 1905b, p. 40). Freud did not stop at this rhetorical interrogation and immediately proceeded that the meaning of a symptom is case-specific. A symptom has therefore no inherent meaning: "In every instance the meaning can be a different one, according to the nature of the suppressed thoughts which are struggling for expression" (Freud 1905b, p. 41). What is interesting about this quote is that the term "diagnosis" is no longer related to an underlying illness. The main thing now is to search for the exact relational context and specific aspects of the experiences of the patient that are linked psychologically with the symptom. The underlying idea is that a symptom is only known thoroughly when we have a clear overview of the ideas that the patient links explicitly or implicitly associatively to it.

This shift in the use of the term "diagnosis" does not imply that Freud would no longer use the term to refer to forms of psychopathology. The most important thing is that he broadens the diagnostic task with it. Making a diagnosis is clearly much more than classifying patients in nosological categories. The singular manifestation of a problem and the question about the status or the function of a problem in a person's life is now identified as an indispensable diagnostic focal point. In fact, far more important than the question of the precise category in which a patient is classified is the question of the entire dynamics of functioning in which problems are embedded.

Such an approach to diagnosis emphasizes the *function* of the symptom and treats each psychological problem as a person-specific construction.[1] The result is that this form of diagnosis is by necessity casuistic. The main

---

[1] In addition, I might add that Freud distinguishes two major components in the symptom: a meaning-related component and a satisfaction-related component. With the meaning-related component, he refers to the idea that behind a specific symptom often lurks a whole story about issues that are either too painful or too difficult to express. Formulated using the distinction between the signifier and the signified, this means that symptoms express a signified that was displaced or could not be articulated otherwise. The symptom itself is a signifier referring to this signified. The signified in question can only be understood by taking the symptom as a signifier and bringing it into dialog with other signifiers. On the other hand, according to Freud the symptom also implies a satisfaction-related component. The symptom affects the person who has the symptom, and in his turmoil it shows itself to be a form of gratification. The satisfaction is excessive, and as a result she cannot recognize it. Psychoanalytic theory on this satisfaction-related component of the symptom is complex, but an example can lift a tip of the veil. When we must stay in bed because we have flu, we feel like a victim of symptoms (e.g., headaches, muscle pain, chills) that we can only control with rest and fever inhibitors. The illness therefore temporarily gives us a condition of suffering. Yet, because we are the victims of flu, we also temporarily receive a number of advantages handed out to us (e.g., we do not have to work and people around us take extra care of us). This "illness benefit" is an aspect of the satisfaction that symptoms carry with them.

thing is the *subjective logic* in someone's functioning. The diagnostician has the task of grasping and describing this very precisely. Concretely this gives rise to case formulation or case construction. Disorder-targeted checklist diagnosis flows into the process of giving a disorder its label. Function-oriented diagnosis, by contrast, generates an *organized narrative*: a statement that articulates how someone's functioning and dysfunctioning are organized. Indeed, at the center of a function-oriented approach to diagnosis is the question concerning the way in which a person's problems are embedded in her wider functioning. Within this view the symptom is a signifier to which signifieds are connected that shift with the context.

The basis for the content of a case formulation consists of material from clinical meetings, such as conversation material from sessions, observations collected in a hospital unit, or data from psychological testing. In a case formulation, a diagnostician discusses this material with the aim of expressing *how* problems are organized. Theory is necessary for building such a case construction, which implies that different theories most probably result in different kinds of explanation. Characteristically, when considering a specific symptom a behavioral therapist will focus on learning processes; a psychoanalyst on the status of the unconscious, and a family therapist on relationship dynamics. Theory is used in this context to read the material and to comprehend something of its complexity. Indeed, theory must act as a compass, but it is pointless if the concepts become a straitjacket into which the patient must fit.

By focusing so strongly on a casuistic description the concern can arise that with such a function-oriented approach all comparability goes adrift. This is mistaken. A function-oriented approach allows us to aggregate information about symptoms at a group level, and enables a bottom-up mapping of how symptoms are interrelated. In line with Borsboom (Borsboom et al. 2011; Borsboom and Cramer 2013) and Van Os (2010; Wigman et al. 2013) I believe that patterns of symptom aggregation provide a much clearer picture about forms of psychopathology than the DSM could ever offer. Since the function-oriented approach puts a great emphasis on the symptom, it is certainly very important for future psychopathology research to become more focused on defining and distinguishing kinds of psychological symptoms, and on studying the way in which symptoms change over time and through interventions.

Case Construction

Since the early days of psychotherapy, case constructions have been used to understand how someone's problems are organized. Freud can be considered as the person who developed the first psychotherapeutic case formulations, together with Freud and Breuer (1895). In the meantime, of course, a great deal has changed. For example, out of dissatisfaction with the purely classificatory approach to psychological problems within the field of psychiatry, behavioral therapists created the methodology of behavioral analysis (Kanfer and Saslow 1965), and in the wake of Carl Rogers, client-oriented psychotherapists began to work with case formulations (Faber, Brink and Raskin 1996).

On the basis of an overview study of definitions that authors with various theoretical backgrounds use, in this regard, Sturmey states (2009, p. 8) that a case formulation usually has the following four characteristics:

1. It discusses the core aspects of a case; that is, it does not just list endless details about the patient and the content of sessions.
2. A case formulation integrates the information about a case in the context of a coherent idea about the nature of the problems with which the patient is struggling.
3. Case formulations are always tentative and reflect what the clinician knows until then. In other words, additional information may always ensure that one can revise her opinion about a case.
4. A case formulation aims at giving direction to the treatment.

These characteristics indicate that a case formulation is a *reasoned assumption*. The diagnostician starts by listening and observing—sometimes supplemented with test results—and brings the gathered information into dialog with theoretical ideas and research data on psychopathological mechanisms and structures. In this interplay between clinical material and theoretical knowledge the diagnostician, making use of abductive reasoning, constructs a logical-plausible hypothesis about how an individual's problems are organized. The work on a case formulation consists of a continuous dialectic between the collection of clinical data and a theoretically informed reading of the collected material. Along this path the diagnostician constructs a knowledgeable and relevant interpretation of the individual's (dys)functioning, without assuming that they can ever provide an exactly correct explanation. Case formulations articulate a plausible construction, but the explanation is never complete. The knowledge that we build along this path is uncertain and not to be simply generalized to other cases or over time. Think of Freud's (1905) remark about aphony: with his patient Dora this symptom was connected to the absence of her beloved at the time of the therapy, but nothing guarantees that this will be true for other patients. Moreover, there is nothing to ensure that any subsequent episodes of aphony with the same patient would again be connected to the absence of a loved one. Note that a case construction is usually built up on the basis of material that is collected in a limited time period. They are not longitudinal observations that reflect the actual path through which a symptom has evolved, but information that at most expresses logical relations between specific aspects of someone's functioning. That is why it is also usually not justified to draw causal conclusions in a case construction. What can be achieved at best is a clarification of the internal structure in someone's functioning. At the same time, clinical case constructions should be more than just psychological snapshots, and integrate information about the symptom in a time frame that characterizes its genesis as well as evolution across time.

Given the tentative nature of a case formulation is it possible that two diagnosticians interpret the functioning of a patient in different ways, particularly when they use different theoretical frameworks. In addition, both constructions can be pertinent and articulate a plausible framework around the problems someone is wrestling with. In order to determine what formulation is the best, one needs to take a pragmatic position: The value of a case formulation depends on the extent to which it enables the clinician to respond adequately.

Qualitative Research as a Methodological Framework

Through its strong focus on a casuistic study of the subjective logic in a patient's functioning this kind of diagnosis is by itself a vulnerable method: vulnerable, that is, to becoming too strongly influenced by the style of a diagnostician, and by errors of thinking or preconceptions in her functioning. That is why we link our plea for function-oriented diagnosis by means of case formulation to the need to also systematize clearly this form of clinical diagnosis. Good function-oriented case formulation entails a method for quality monitoring that helps diagnosticians to optimize the validity and reliability of their decision-making.

To articulate principles for quality control, literature about the methodology of qualitative research is most useful. Obviously, clinical case formulation cannot just be considered as a form of qualitative research. Clinical casuistry aims at formulating a good and usable characterization of problems and strengths in someone's functioning, and is often constructed while working with an individual: through clinical meetings (discussions, observations, testing) material is collected, and while doing so ideas are constructed concerning the organization of someone's (dys)functioning. The time spent in building a case formulation is usually considerably less than the time spent on the actual clinical contact. Qualitative research on the other hand often has a more generalizing focus and aims at building controlled knowledge that carries much further than the personal situation of the participants. In order to achieve this type of knowledge one works with time-intensive forms of data analysis, which usually take much more time than the data collection.

Furthermore, in the context of psychiatric diagnosis *questions* and *knowledge* have another status. Typically, qualitative research starts with a question of the researcher: something in the outside world intrigues her and starting from this question she aims to build an explanation. The researcher hopes to construct knowledge to help others understand how an aspect of reality is organized. An example of such a qualitative study is found in the work of Nicole Highet and colleagues (2014). In collaboration with colleagues she examined how post-natal depression and post-natal anxiety are embedded into the world of women who are struggling with such experiences. On the basis of 28 interviews she discerns that experiences of loss and frustration appear to be at the basis of these forms of anxiety and depression. Herewith she points to the role of pregnancy-related changes (such as the change of one's body shape) and disappointments that go hand in hand with pregnancy and maternity (such as complications with childbirth or conflicts around parenting with the partner). Such studies construct knowledge that is to be generalized beyond the specific situation of the women from the research sample. The researchers try to formulate insights that sharpen our general understanding about a specific aspect of psychological functioning. In clinical diagnostic situations, by contrast, the person who consults the psy-professional asks the question. The patient suffers from how she functions and at that point would like help from a professional, with the hope that eventually the disturbing component will be resolved. The knowledge that the diagnostician builds aims at clarifying the problem and the experience, such that relevant interventions may be organized. The knowledge of the diagnostician does not involve the construction of generalizable knowledge. It is a practically oriented form of knowing that aims to clarify the structure or dynamic of one's actions. For example, suppose that a young woman consults because of lethargy after the birth of a second child. General knowledge of post-natal mood problems, as found in the study of Highet et al. (2014), may be useful in this context as a background, but it is not enough to know what is going on. Only by learning in great detail about the mental and relational world of the woman in question can we see how the problem is embedded in her life and in her speech. The knowledge that a diagnostician constructs along this way has a strong singular component that is usually filtered out in scientific research: specificities that apply to this one individual stand to the fore.

What the work with clinical case formulations and qualitative research clearly have in common is a focus on language and speaking on the one hand, and an explicit emphasis on constructing well-reasoned assumptions about someone's functioning on the other hand. Methodological guidelines concerning qualitative research can never simply be imposed on clinical diagnostic work, but can help to improve the quality of work with case formulations. It is in this way that I propose using them. Since case formulation primarily focuses on the nature and underlying structure of someone's experience, we can place it in the field of the qualitative inquiry.

In the heyday of positivistic approaches in psychology (during the second half of the twentieth century) qualitative research was marginalized. Starting from the idea that only numerical data could form the basis of science, the value of narratives and non-quantitative observation data was disregarded for a long time.

However, qualitative research has a long history and had a place in psychology from the beginning. For example, Wilhelm Wundt (1897), one of the founders of experimental psychology, claimed that we must distinguish two research approaches. On the one hand Wundt distinguishes experimental psychology, which deals with the study of specific psychological functions, such as perception, memory, or cognition, and starts from laboratory studies following the model of the natural sciences. Within this paradigm the human *psyche* is seen as an object that one tries to access with exact measuring instruments. The subjective experience of the individual is ignored in such an approach. On the other hand, Wundt also discerns a branch of research that focuses on the study of so-called higher mental processes, such as the way in which a person interprets and experiences the world. Wundt indicates that such an approach to mental processes should make up the actual focus of psychology, and starts from interpretative research strategies that tally with what we now call qualitative methods.[2]

For a long time, the systematic study of subjective experience was barely part of psychological research. Many years empirical and rationalist approaches dominated the question of how humans function, and as a result there was little room for the question of how subjective experience is organized (Bruner 1990, 1991; Lacan 1959; Merleau-Ponty 1945). For years psychologists mainly thought mechanically about the human experience, as if humans were a complex machine or a computer in which the hardware and the software could be studied in detail. Whereas in the eighteenth century the French philosopher Julien Offray de la Mettrie (1747) was ostracized because in his essay "L'homme machine" he dared

---

[2] Note that other pioneers from psychology, such as William James, William Stern, Lev Vygotski, and Leon Festinger, have also made a similar distinction (Marecek 2003).

to say that the human mind as well as the human body functions according to mechanistic natural laws, in the twentieth century it suddenly appeared pseudoscientific *not* to look at the human being as an ingenious machine. Qualitative research, as we know it now, was shaped out of a dissatisfaction with such mechanistic thinking and focuses on the study of subjectivity in particular (Madill and Gough 2008). Conversely, for a long time many academics and practitioners from the clinical field plainly neglected the question of the scientificity of their work. Wundt's suggestion to develop appropriate methods for the systematic study of subjectivity remained unheard and did not reach the clinic. Scientific evaluation was only too happily left to the discretion of the laboratory psychologist working at a safe distance. Yet in the past decades attitudes have changed. In the nerve center of psychology, space for qualitative approaches was made, which aimed to study subjectivity following stringent methodological guidelines.

Jerome Bruner was one of the leading figures that very clearly made a plea for qualitative approaches in psychology. Bruner was partly at the origin of the so-called cognitive revolution. Out of dissatisfaction with the black-box approach of the behaviorist movement, which did not want to be involved with the study of internal psychological processes, he appealed to colleagues for an approach to human beings as generators of meaning. However, fairly early on he observed that within the cognitive movement all attention was being given to the way people *process* information, while the question as to *how* they make sense of themselves and the world disappeared into the background. Going against this tendency, Bruner (1990, 1991) argued that human beings should be considered as cultural creatures that produce narrative truths. Through language, humans structure the world:

> We organize our experience and our memory of human happenings mainly in the form of narrative—stories, excuses, myths, reasons for doing and not doing, and so on. Narrative is a conventional form, transmitted culturally and constrained by each individual's level of mastery and by his conglomerate of prosthetic devices, colleagues, and mentors. Unlike the constructions generated by logical and scientific procedures that can be weeded out by falsification, narrative constructions can only achieve "verisimilitude."

Narratives, then, are a version of reality whose acceptability is governed by convention and "narrative necessity" rather than by empirical verification and logical requiredness. (Bruner 1991, p. 4)

The research that Bruner initiated was not clinically oriented, but his narrative approach connects closely with the work of the diagnostician who builds on case formulation. Indeed, the diagnostician also works with stories. These stories are not only listened to but also explored and synthesized, with the aim of grasping how the patient's account is organized and embedded in broader contexts.

According to Bruner (1990), the psychological study of stories should bring the perspective of the narrator to the fore. Stories never speak for themselves, and always entail a major interpretation component that we have to take into account. To get hold of what a narrative means, Bruner (1991) examines the background from which the narrator speaks.

Applied to case formulation this implies that complaints and problems always need to be studied from the perspective of the person articulating them. Rather than generalize, neutralize, or anonymize complaints by means of diagnostic jargon, a narratively oriented qualitative approach requires us to clearly bring into account their person-specific status and to see how they are socially and culturally embedded (Parker 2005).

One point that stands out in both Bruner's and Wundt's work, and around which qualitative researchers unite more generally, is that the subjectivity of the participant should be central: "The heart of qualitative inquiry is its epistemological stance: its commitment to interrogating subjectivity, intentional action, and experiences embedded in real-life contexts" (Marecek 2003, p. 55). Qualitative psychologists do not want to make universal claims about the way phenomena are organized, but map the diversity and complexity of the human experience: "they are not searching for fundamentals of psychic life that exist apart from social context and they do not seek to make universalized claims about psychic life. Instead they set their sights on the ways in which human action and social identities are locally constituted and contingent on their time and place" (Marecek 2003, pp. 56–57). Furthermore, qualitative researchers consider language as the best way to get in touch with human subjectivity. Rather than rely on a variety of measurement instruments, qualitative researchers study the psychological reality of human beings through natural language use (Polkinghorne 1990). It is precisely by paying attention to subjective experience, diversity, and language use that there is a strong similarity between the focus of the qualitative researcher and that of the diagnostician who works with case formulations.

However, the points of commonality between various qualitative researchers have not given rise to the development of a generally accepted qualitative method, but to a variety of approaches that operate next to each other. Several methods of qualitative inquiry co-exist and often also have different aims (Madill and Gough 2008). For example, a phenomenological researcher who wants to gain insight into the nature and meaning of mental experiences has a very different approach compared to a scholar who (via discourse analysis) aims to grasp how language use reproduces power relationships. This methodological multiplicity offers a variety of perspectives for researchers, but does not foreground one single method of analyzing interview and observation data.

Quality Assurance in Diagnostic Case Formulation

One idea around which more consensus seems to have been reached is that qualitative research is only solid if it passes the critical test of methodological quality criteria. The past few years have seen the publication of overview studies on factors that need to be taken into consideration when monitoring the quality of qualitative research. The underlying idea is that the soundness of scientific research does not depend that much on the type of data that it collects—quantitative or qualitative—but on the methodology used. Scientifically sound research implies that sources that might distort the decision-making process are excluded as much as possible, or controlled for by using systematic reflection.

In what follows I discuss three major points of attention to monitor the quality of qualitative research: *reflexivity, reliability*, and *validity*. Reflexivity is pivotal to good quality assurance, and indicates the need for an overall critical attitude. Reliability relates to the importance of systematic work and to excluding possible sources of distortion.

Validity concerns the efforts to guarantee that findings are correct. With my discussion of these points I will also indicate how they can be applied to diagnostic case formulations. Some readers may be surprised by this great emphasis on quality assurance and by the detailed focus on the methodology of qualitative research. Following the critiques on psychiatric diagnosis, as discussed in Chaps. 2 and 3, I believe that within the practice of clinical diagnosis more attention should be paid to the soundness and accuracy of the processes through which we draw conclusions about people's mental health condition. Diagnostic statements have far-reaching implications (what interventions are or are not taken? Which characteristics are attributed to a person? etc.), and must therefore be well founded and carefully constructed. Most of the methods for quality assurance that I propose are not new. However, often these methods are not integrated into a systematic quality policy and I would appeal for this to be done. Mental health care professionals and organizations would enhance the inherent quality of their diagnostic work and the trustworthiness of their conclusions if they clarify how they optimize the components of reflexivity, reliability, and validity.

Reflexivity

The first point of quality assurance that qualitative researchers pay much attention to is reflexivity. By being aware of the impact of social and cultural contexts, qualitative researchers reflect how they may influence the interpretation process. Just like the people they study, qualitative researchers actively interpret the world they are dealing with. Researchers do not work in a social vacuum but exercise their role against a background (family, training, employment, etc.) that cannot be ignored. Although this is epistemologically naïve, many researchers tend to regard research as an objective and value-free activity (Ponterotto 2005). Qualitative researchers, on the contrary, explicitly start from the idea that each study is loaded with value and thus has a moral dimension: the person of the researcher cannot be excluded from the research process (Malterud 2001).

By paying explicit attention to how they are personally intertwined with their inquiries, qualitative researchers bring into account the influence of values, preferences, and opinions: "reflexivity is a way of *attending to the institutional location of historical and personal aspects of the research relationship*" (Parker 2005, p. 25). Concretely, reflexivity takes shape by reflecting on the way in which a researcher is influenced by the context in which she works. In this way, several layers of influence are distinguished (Malterud 2001; Parker 2005).

There is first and above all the influence of the researcher as a person. The private life, the history, experiences, and ideas of the researcher inevitably have an impact on the decisions they make. The way in which this impact might take shape could be best explained as follows: "Reflexivity starts by identifying preconceptions brought into the project by the researcher, representing previous personal and professional experiences, pre-study beliefs about how things are and what is to be investigated, motivation and qualifications for exploration of the field, and perspectives and theoretical foundations related to education and interests" (Malterud 2001, p. 484). Across the entire research process a good qualitative researcher asks how her own past and present can influence what she perceives and ignores in the studied material. In practice this reflection usually takes shape by using a *research diary*, in which annotations are made about his or her personal interdependence with the project. These notes are a crucial component within the research process and important or remarkable elements of it are often ultimately processed in publications. Sharp reports on the reflexive process clarify how the author makes sense of reality and allows readers to put the position of the researcher into perspective.

The second layer of influence that reflexivity addresses is more structural, and relates to the institutional embedding of the researcher (Parker 2005). Researchers are exponents of a social context that has its own interests, which group members typically reproduce, even if they are not aware of it. For example, a researcher studying how double-income couples with children experience work and family life from the point of view of an employer will most probably highlight other points than a researcher addressing the same question from the point of view of an interest group for families. In the same way education and socialization within a particular discipline or theoretical school of thought also influence what researchers see and hear. In an interview study on the way people experience psychiatric diagnoses, a sociologist will most probably notice things that a psychiatrist would not; on the other hand, a psychoanalyst will conduct the interview differently than a behavioral therapist. In a good research diary the qualitative researcher reflects on these influences with the aim of discussing them in publications.

The third layer of influence concerns the relationship between the researcher and the person examined (Parker 2005). Since the researcher occupies the position of the one who asks questions and aims to formulate ideas through the interaction with a participant, their relationship implies implicit power dynamics. Usually, the researcher occupies a superior position. Take, for example, the study of Temerlin (1968, 1970), in which participants diagnose an actor. With some participants an eminent colleague makes a remark about the interview, while with other participants this is not the case. Within this design the participant is subject to experimental manipulation, while the researcher keeps control. The researcher is also the one who gains the knowledge that the experiment produces: Temerlin publishes *his* insights about how the participants behave and explains why they act in this way. Within such a design participants are expected to participate in an obedient way but will not personally acquire any knowledge through their participation in such a study. This creates a balance of power that is similar to the one Foucault (1973–1974) detects between a diagnostician and patient. Researchers deem problems relevant because they have knowledge about certain phenomena and the privilege of this knowledge is precisely what determines the power imbalance ('Knowledge is power!' as the sixteenth-century humanist Francis Bacon proclaimed). Qualitative researchers therefore explicitly ask how their knowledge position creates a power imbalance and examine how they can counter the negative impact of this imbalance. In order to avoid a power imbalance they might, for example, prefer the method of participant observation, which creates minimal interference with how people usually act and behave. What is more, research participants may not only be actively involved with the data collection, but may also be given a role in the decision-making process of a study. Again, the research diary is a good instrument to report on such questions and to search for relevant solutions.

Summarized: reflexivity aims at bringing into account the influence of the researcher (personal, institutional, relational) on the investigation process. Through reflection in a research diary the researcher can actively try to avoid unwanted influences, and give others access to the perspective from which she is collecting data and interpreting the world.

An interesting addition to the idea of reflexivity is found in the work of the French anthropologist Claude Lévi-Strauss. In his pioneering study on structural anthropology Lévi-Strauss (1958) suggests that we must not simply identify the influence emanating from the person and the context of the researcher, but should also rule it out as much as possible. In order to get acquainted with the otherness of the other, that is, with the dimension of the Other, you need to forget yourself enough in order to be able to attend to what the Other says and does not say. According to Lévi-Strauss (1958, p. 118) this can only be realized if the researcher actively applies the so-called *technique de dépaysement*. This means that when thinking about culture the anthropologist cultivates a position of marginality, and puts his own ideas about the world between brackets as much as possible. By becoming marginal with respect to what is evident (your own culture), possibilities open up to develop a more unprejudiced and subtle approach to what is strange (the other culture). Through such methodological marginalization the researcher acquires a particularly appropriate strategy to get hold of the otherness of the other: "In the social sciences the person of the researcher is the only instrument to gain knowledge of human behaviour; the primary access to the thoughts and the actions of others. This is why this splitting of identity [by means of the *technique de dépaysement*] is epistemologically so important: it enables a self-disciplining of the gaze, meaning a methodical putting into brackets of an important dimension of subjectivity" (Lemaire 2008, p. 27). What Lévi-Strauss's principle of cultivating a position of marginality adds is that reflexivity should not remain stuck at a cognitive level. Cultivating a position of marginality implies that the researcher develops an attitude of open-mindedness and tries to exclude the influence of many preconceptions.

Reflexivity in the Context of Function-Oriented Case Formulation

Applied to the praxis of clinical case construction, reflexivity implies that in preparing case formulations diagnosticians should bring into account the influence of their own perspective. Indeed, consistent with the epistemological symptom model of Marková and Berrios (2009), clinicians should not be thought of as objective observers. Therefore it is of the utmost importance that within the process of diagnosis, personal and contextual influences from the diagnostician are kept in check as well as possible. By having an adequate idea of the influence the clinician brings into the diagnostic processes, the singularity of the patient can be central, which manages the potential bias outlined by Meehl (1973).

In order to adequately get hold of the problems someone suffers from, and to contextualize them in terms of the other's position in the world, diagnosticians should be sufficiently marginalized from what they believe is self-evident. This is an important basic principle. Lacan (1956a, p. 394) underscores this by stating that the clinician should "beware of understanding" (Lacan 1956a, p. 471). Whoever tries to understand the experiences and words of the Other from the background of own ideas and experiences takes herself too strongly as a criterion. Deliberate non-understanding makes the clinician alert for the unexpected. The underlying idea is that those who do not yet understand pay more attention to what the other person says and does, and therefore also get a better hold of the new. In parallel with what Lévi-Strauss indicates about the anthropologist, a diagnostician must, according to Lacan, be sufficiently marginalized of what she thinks is obvious and normal. Just as the *technique de dépaysement, gardez-vous de comprendre* forms not only a methodological but also an ethical basic principle. It implies a position of respect for the otherness of the other. Through their decisions diagnosticians inevitably intervene within the lives of others, in that clinical work always has an unmistakable ethical dimension: "No clinic without ethics" (Miller 1983, p. 65).

Deliberate non-understanding provides a good starting point for reflexive clinical work, but to practically give shape to reflexivity the clinician might find inspiration in the approach of the qualitative researcher, and take into account the three layers of influence (personal, institutional, relational) that the attitude of reflexivity builds upon.

Personal reflexivity then means that one takes into account how the diagnostician is involved in, and is affected by, the process of diagnosis. Above all, a diagnostician acts as a professional, but next to that she is affected by a continuous flow of thoughts and impulses. In making professional decisions she is inevitably influenced by memories and previous experiences, as well as her own likes and dislikes. Such an influence cannot be ruled out. It is therefore important that the clinician consider *how* this influence affects her. In this way a biased attitude can be avoided. It is only by remaining open to the way in which patients affect us that we can keep our spontaneous preconceptions at a distance and ensure that diagnostic judgment is influenced by our own peculiarities as little as possible.

An example of such a reflexive preparation is found with Freud. In the beginning of his psychoanalytic career Freud published three books in which reflections on his own impulses and thoughts are central: *The Interpretation of Dreams* (Freud 1900), *Psychopathology of Everyday Life* (Freud 1901), and *The Joke and Its Relationship with the Unconscious* (Freud 1905a). In these books Freud examines, on the one hand, material that he collected with other people. On the other hand, he also scrutinizes his own functioning, asking why he has certain dreams, makes mistakes of a particular kind, or finds certain jokes amusing. What is characteristic for *The Interpretation of Dreams* is that he thinks of dreams as puzzles, and searches how his wider lines of thought are associatively linked to the manifest dream content. What is interesting here in terms of our examination of reflexivity is that as a result of certain dreams Freud also writes about his clinical work, and through his associations reaches thoughts that do not comply with his professional starting position. A clear illustration of this is found in his (1900, pp. 124–137) dream about his previous patient Anna Hammerslag (Fichtner 2010), whom he gave the name Irma in *The Interpretation of Dreams*. The stimulus for the dream was feedback from a colleague that Anna Hammerslag was in a bad condition. Freud was upset and took it upon himself to write out the disease history of this patient. That night he had a dream about her, in which she makes it clear to him that she still feels pain.[3] In the dream Freud then examines the patient's throat with colleagues and concludes that an erroneous intervention of another doctor must be the source of her condition. In *The Interpretation of Dreams* Freud explores the broader ideas that various parts of the dream are connected with, and examines what the dream brings to mind. Along this way, a component of reproach in relation to the patient and his fellow doctors comes to the fore. Concerns and feelings of guilt about his own state of health, private family members, Anna Hammerslag, and other patients also appear, as well as a very brief sexual idea. Historically speaking, Freud's dream book is innovative because he is not hesitating to assess the impact of the clinical work on his subjectivity. "No one who, like me, conjures up the most evil of those half-tamed demons that inhabit the human breast, and seeks to wrestle with them, can expect to come through the struggle unscathed" (Freud 1905b, p. 109). Clinical work never leaves the clinician unaffected. Yet in order to prevent this from becoming the guideline of clinical intervention, the clinician must learn to look at the impact that this kind of work has on herself, and also any personal prejudice she may allow into her professional activity. According to Freud, such subjective influences can only be controlled for by reflecting openly and by exploring how working

---

[3] The entire dream goes as follows: "A large hall—numerous guests, whom we were receiving. -Among them was Irma. I at once took her on one side, as though to answer her letter and to reproach her for not having accepted my 'solution' yet. I said to her: 'If you still get pains, it's really only your fault.' She replied: 'If you only knew what pains I've got now in my throat and stomach and abdomen—it's choking me'—I was alarmed and looked at her. She looked pale and puffy. I thought to myself that after all I must be missing some organic trouble. I took her to the window and looked down her throat, and she showed signs of recalcitrance, like women with artificial dentures. I thought to myself that there was really no need for her to do that.—She then opened her mouth properly and on the right I found a big white patch; at another place I saw extensive whitish grey scabs upon some remarkable curly structures which were evidently modelled on the turbinal bones of the nose.—I at once called in Dr. M., and he repeated the examination and confirmed it. … Dr M. looked quite different from usual; he was very pale, he walked with a limp and his chin was clean-shaven. … My friend Otto was now standing beside her as well, and my friend Leopold was percussing her through her bodice and saying: 'She has a dull area low down on her left.' He also indicated that a portion of the skin on the left shoulder was infiltrated. (I noticed this, just as he did, in spite of her dress.). … M. said 'There's no doubt its an infection, but no matter; dysentery will supervene and the toxin will eliminated.' … We were directly aware, too, of the origin of her infection. Not long before, when she was feeling unwell, my friend Otto had given her an injection of a preparation of propyl, propyls … propionic acid … trimethylamin (and I saw before me the formula for this printed in heavy type). … Injections of that sort ought not to be made so thoughtlessly. … And probably the syringe had not been clean" (Freud 1900, p. 107).

with patients affects the clinician (i.e., by provoking memories, anger or fear, daydreaming, a desire for friendship, etc.). It brings the clinician to consider sensitive situations with a meta-perspective. This is extremely important for the patient: by filtering out the subjective influence, the diagnostician can keep the patient central in the work. This is also very important for the clinician herself. Studies of professional burnout suggest that occupying a meta-perspective is characteristic for professionals who are not burned out (Vanheule et al. 2003; Vanheule and Verhaeghe 2004).

The *institutional embedding* of the diagnostician represents the second layer of influence that reflexivity addresses. Psy-professionals, just like (qualitative) researchers, never work in a social vacuum and must ensure that they monitor the influence that results from the position they occupy in social groups. Indeed, diagnosticians are trained and socialized within specific schools of thought about diagnosis, and more broadly different models of psychopathology. For example, the distinction between disorder-oriented classificatory diagnosis and function-oriented case formulation represents two schools of thought on diagnosis. When diagnosing, one cannot but start from such a frame. A theoretical framework is needed to bring order to the multitude of raw material the clinician collects. Obviously, this does not preclude the importance of looking at such theories from a distance. While constructing a case formulation the patient must be central, not the theory. When the theory is central, we run the risk of ending up in what Verhaeghe (2002) calls *paradigmatic thinking*. This means that one applies theory dogmatically and behaves like the good student who expects approval from his teacher. Such a use of theory benefits only the narcissism of a diagnostician. By addressing cases as illustrations of a certain theory, one puts oneself in the light of the master, thus enjoying the genius one hopes to share with the master. In terms of group dynamics, paradigmatic thinking creates cohesion, but what is lost is the dimension of deliberate non-understanding. Verhaeghe formulates this as follows (2002, p. 72): "the paradigm's real function is to create nest warmth, that is to say, to offer an articulated and hence security-providing framework for its followers, collected around a central credo that supplies a comforting answer to the ever-threatening Real of the clinic." Reflexive work implies that the diagnostician avoids the paradigmatic application of theory and models as much as possible and at the same time also clearly communicates on the theoretical points of departure that orient the diagnosis.

In addition to this influence of theory at an institutional level, the work of the context of the diagnostician also has a major influence, just like the zeitgeist within which he/she is working. For example, professionals employed in social work settings (where traditionally much attention is paid to context) will naturally look at problems differently to someone who works in a rehabilitation center (where traditionally attention is paid to individual-specific disorder characteristics). For a child that ends up in one or the other sector it is possible that such a work context entails a different diagnostic focus. Reflexive work implies that the diagnostician is clearly aware of such influence and communicates on the implicit assumptions that are taken for granted in the sector or organization in which they work. It is only by making these assumptions explicit that one can have an eye and an ear for their limitations.

As regards the influence of the zeitgeist, the phenomenon of diagnostic trends is important. The history of psychiatry and psychology shows that over time there have always been diagnoses that are fashionable for a while, and are therefore given en mass (Showalter 1998). Just as certain theories may lead to narrow paradigmatic thinking, diagnostic trends can also function as a Procrustean bed where everyone, reluctant or not, must fit in. Once the unfounded nature of fashionable diagnoses come to light, rebutting these seems easy. Yet, what is trendy should not be used as a benchmark. This is the actual challenge. A reflexive attitude toward diagnosis should bring the clinician to detecting diagnostic trends, and to take into account her own susceptibility to such trends.

The relationship between the diagnostician and the diagnosed person is the third layer of influence that we can distinguish in reflexivity. In Chap. 2 we noted that in line with Foucault (1973–1974) power dynamics may be discerned in the relationship between clinician and patient. Psychiatric power is established since knowledge plays a particular role in the diagnostic process. The diagnostician has power because people expect that the psy-professional can adequately assess what their problem is. It is presumed that the diagnostician holds the truth about someone's functioning. Indeed, diagnostic power takes shape because in the diagnostic situation submission to the knowledgeable diagnostician is taken for granted: "it is the patient's own account that constitutes the moment when the truth blazes forth" (Foucault 1973–1974, p. 11). Moreover Foucault suggests that typically mental health care services are organized such that power is consolidated again and again: through common interactions, institutions subject the patient to the professional's working regime. For example, this is reflected in rules concerning access to meetings and to files, or in the fact that the patient has to remain in the waiting room until the clinician calls her (Foucault 1973–1974).

Within the context of anti-psychiatry, analyses of power dynamics have sometimes led to a rejection of the entire psy-establishment, as if psychological problems are only an effect of social structures brought into being by psy-professionals. Assuming that mental suffering has a real basis, such a rejection is not very relevant. However, Foucault's analysis alerts us to the inherent presence of power within diagnostic relationships. Instead of wanting to eliminate this dimension of power, it is more relevant to deal with it correctly in a constructive and ethical manner. In this context Lacan (1961) suggests that the professional should not use the power attributed to her to guide the patient in a particular direction, but use it to bring the patient's subjective truth to the fore. Indeed, the diagnostic situation should be organized such that the otherness of the other is brought to the fore.

Dealing with diagnostic power in a reflexive way firstly implies that one acts such that the person asking for help is enabled and empowered in bringing her subjective truth to the fore. On the other hand, it implies that a diagnostician questions herself about the influence emanating from the professional status attributed to her as a psy-professional.

In line with this distinction between the three layers of influence, we can ask the question for appropriate methods to give shape to reflexivity in practice. Indeed, clinicians should not only pay lip service to the idea of reflexivity but implement it effectively and explicitly in their diagnostic work by using work formats that ensure the accomplishment of critical reflection.

In Freud's work we already encountered the first idea on how reflexivity can take shape: by analyzing his dreams, Freud investigates how clinical work affects him. Sustained self-analysis is important, but other methods for implementing reflexivity should be considered as well. Whether someone engages in self-analysis or not is largely a personal matter. It contributes to enhancing the quality of the clinical work but strongly depends on the dedication of the individual clinician. In a similar vein, committing oneself to a personal psychoanalysis or some form of psychotherapy might provide unparalleled opportunities for reflection on the position one occupies as a diagnostician,[4] but it is unlikely that every psy-professional is willing to commit to such endeavor. In mental health care settings self-analysis and engagement in a personal psychoanalysis or psychotherapy cannot be implemented structurally to give shape to reflexivity.

One method for the promotion of reflexivity consistent with self-analysis, and a kind of variation on the research diary of the qualitative researcher, is the *clinical diary*. Qualitative researchers use a research diary to write down daily thoughts and remarks about a research project. Along this way they can check how they are personally involved in the project: "Researchers are expected to reflect on how they come to know what they know, and the chronicle of one's thinking contained in a research journal potentially facilitates such awareness" (Watt 2007, p. 96). Writing supports a thinking process that allows the researcher to better contain the complexity of the investigation: "Writing is also a way of 'knowing'—a method of discovery and analysis. By writing in different ways, we discover new aspects of our topic and our relationship to it" (Richardson 1994, p. 516). In the same vein, the clinical diary is an interesting thinking instrument for the diagnostician. Whoever works with patients will, on the one hand, collect patient-oriented working notes. These contain notations about (dynamics in) the functioning of the patient. A clinical

---

[4] These are normally part of the formation process for psychoanalysts and psychotherapists. Lacan indicates that the purposes of a personal psychoanalysis for a psychoanalyst (sometimes called "didactical analysis") consist of learning to recognize and conquer the "alienation in relation to oneself"—*aliénation à vous-même* (Lacan 1956b, p. 161). The idea of "alienation in relation to oneself" points to an obstinate hanging-on to the image of oneself; to ideas, values … in relation to others. Whoever puts the image of oneself as central has the tendency to also treat this own self-image as the standard to judge others, for example when one makes a judgment about what is normal and what is not. A personal psychoanalysis has the objective of enabling the candidate-psychoanalyst to leave behind his blindness and deafness, so that in the clinical work one learns to listen to what others actually say: "if didactical psychoanalysis makes sense, it is to make you hear yourself respond to the subject, so that you know what he tells you" (Lacan 1956b, p. 161).

diary has another function, and is prepared from personal notes. It is a document in which the clinician writes down thoughts and concerns about her general way of working, about her own particular preferences when working with certain patients, about how she is personally affected by certain situations—or remains unaffected by them—and much more. By writing such a diary and re-reading it, the clinician creates a reflexive distance with respect to her work, and can become aware of what she personally brings to it. A clinical diary can never serve as an alternative to a personal psychoanalysis or psychotherapy, but might encourage the clinician to question the beaten track of her own actions and to consider options for a different approach to the clinic. An interesting example of a clinical diary is found in the work of the Hungarian psychoanalyst Sándor Ferenczi (1995). During his career Ferenczi strongly experimented with all kinds of therapeutic techniques. At the same time, he was very critical of the results he obtained and questioned himself in his diary about his own motivations, which shows reflexivity. An unmistakable restriction linked with keeping a clinical diary, however, is that this form of work is purely based on self-reflection. It is possible that one therefore continues to have difficulty overcoming certain blind spots in one's own thinking.

Supervision, work discussions, and *clinical cartels* are three other methods through which reflexivity could be implemented in practice. Common to these methods is that they build on interactions with others and therefore don't purely consist of self-reflection. This is important because it is precisely by articulating to *another* how we work that we create an aspect of reflexivity that escapes the circles in which our thoughts run. The silence or the punctuation of the other offers the professional opportunities to test and challenge one's own reasoning. In the three methods we discuss below, the interaction enables the construction of some form of knowing. All three facilitate reflective speaking and they engender a dialog around hot topics. Supervision, work discussions, and clinical cartels usually start from concrete cases or incidents, with the aim of constructing the logic that governs the case. Exchanging ideas and hypotheses about the nature of a patient's problem, and how to approach it, is central. These methods can also be used to reflect on the way in which the clinical decision-making process is controlled by the three layers of influence (personal, institutional, relational) that are inherent to the actions of the clinician.

Each of the three methods creates a secure environment to openly and regularly question our own functioning. Research with psychotherapists shows that effective therapists are open to perspective-widening input from others, and also talk directly about their thinking and actions (Miller et al. 2007). Supervision, working discussions, and clinical cartels facilitate both aspects.

More concretely, supervision consists of a series of discussions where one talks with an experienced colleague (supervisor), who is also sufficiently independent of one's own work situation, and focuses on concrete dilemmas, crises, and uncertainties about the work (Bradley 2008). During supervision, questions about the logic of a case and how this is best handled clinically are addressed. In addition, supervision can also focus on the impact of clinical work on the clinician, or on the influence of private issues on her professional actions. Supervision can take place in groups or individually, and always has the objective of shedding light on situations that one does not have a clear view on. Although the word "supervising"[5] etymologically refers to the inspection of whether someone's work has been carried out properly (Harper 2012), this is not explicitly the aim of supervision. As an instrument for reflexivity, it particularly aims to be a form of meta-listening whereby one reorganizes existing material in function of a better understanding of the case. Review studies show that it is a form of work that clinicians experience as supportive (Mor Barak et al. 2009), and that also leads to better clinical decision-making (Farnan et al. 2012).

Work discussion[6] consists of regular consultations between a small and stable group of colleagues, where one meets without superiors and reflects on cases or work-related questions. Through specific clinical material, concerns and issues at work are discussed with the aim of finding new and better ways of approaching or managing a problem: "the task of the group as a whole is to be supportive of a process that will involve a fresh

---

[5] Lacan (1975, p. 42) suggests that we should talk about *super-audition* instead of *supervision*. After all, what is central in this clinical activity is listening and speaking and not so much looking and being looked at.

[6] Sometimes work discussions are referred to with the notion intervision. "Intervision" is, however, a broader term that is used for groups in which intercollegial discussion is central, but in which one does not always work with a discussion leader (Hendriksen 2009).

consideration of what may have been hitherto held rather unquestioningly" (Bradley 2008, p. 23). In contrast to supervision this does not take place in dialog with an experienced outsider; it is group reflection together with people who exercise a similar job, with equal opportunities for each member to participate. Often, work discussions make use of a discussion leader, who has the task of guiding the process and ensuring a good working climate (Bradley 2008). *Balint groups* are an example of a work discussion group. The Balint group method was created by Michael Balint (1957) and lets doctors reflect on dilemmas from the patient-physician relationship and about the emotional impact of their job on the basis of cases from their practice (Van Roy et al. 2014).

Clinical cartels, in their turn, are small work and study groups consisting of four to six people who, over the period of a year, without a supervisor, collaborate intensively around the same subject. In a clinical cartel these are usually cases. Cartels were created by Lacan (1964) to promote a form of reflection and collaboration that is not geared to the opinion of an expert or leader. In order to ensure that all members of the cartel make an active contribution, the group is kept sufficiently small. To ensure commitment of its members, it is further demanded that they achieve a product, such as a written case in lieu of the joint work. In a cartel there is also always one member, the so-called *plus un*, with a special task. On the one hand, this person is working actively with the other members of the cartel, but on the other hand the *plus un* is also responsible for process monitoring. The *plus un* has a task to ensure that all the members of the cartel effectively participate. In addition, she shall ensure that no one dominates the group process, and safeguards that the cartel moves toward the development of an outcome product.

Aiming at Validity and Reliability: A Matter of Careful Verification

By addressing reflexivity a (self-)critical component is built into the clinical work. The principles and work methods presented above encourage the clinician to think, speak, and write about the possible impact of personal, institutional, and relational factors on the diagnostic decision-making process. Implementing reflexivity in routine work practice is important since, in this way, the impact of the clinician and her context on diagnostic decision-making is articulated and explored. By articulating this impact one can ensure that the singularity of the case is always again central in the diagnosis.

Aiming at reliability and validity is complementary to this, and attempts to ensure transparent and correct decision-making. The concepts of reliability and validity originate from the psychometric research tradition, but are also used in qualitative research (Franklin and Ballan 2001; Miles and Huberman 1994; Morse et al. 2002; Golafshani 2003; Stiles 1993). It is important here that validity and reliability are not regarded as static concepts but as processes that require continual attention. Qualitative methods such as open interviews and discussions, through which one studies phenomena in a naturalistic way, are very difficult to standardize. They require an approach to validity and reliability that mainly focuses on the stringency of methodological decision-making.

Such rigor is achieved by paying sufficient attention to *verification* in the process of investigation. This means that one systematically checks whether the decision-making process is operating properly: "Verification is the process of checking, confirming, making sure, and being certain. In qualitative research, verification refers to the mechanisms used during the process of research to incrementally contribute to ensuring reliability and validity and, thus, the rigor of a study" (Morse et al. 2002, p. 9). Verification is linked to a cyclical or iterative approach to research: "a good qualitative researcher moves back and forth between design and implementation to ensure congruence among question formulation, literature, recruitment, data collection strategies, and analysis. Data are systematically checked, focus is maintained, and the fit of data and the conceptual work of analysis and interpretation are monitored and confirmed constantly" (Morse et al. 2002, p. 10). In other words, proper qualitative research requires a good researcher. That is to say: someone who is focused on collecting sufficiently significant material that reflects the studied phenomenon as closely as possible, who pays attention to important details and broader outlines in the material, who draws careful conclusions from the data and uses theory as a lens to read and interpret refined data: "In this way, it is essential that the investigator remain open, use sensitivity, creativity and insight, and be willing to relinquish any ideas that are poorly supported regardless of the excitement and the potential that they first appear to provide. It is these investigator qualities or actions that produce social inquiry and are crucial to the attainment of optimal reliability and validity" (Morse et al. 2002, p. 11). From a qualitative point of view validity and reliability are not standards against which research results are checked once the data are analyzed, but principles one pays attention to throughout the entire research cycle.

The principle of verification is also useful in the context of case formulation-based clinical diagnosis. To come to sound decisions, the clinician must carefully test and check whether conclusions are well founded in the interview material and observation data. Case constructions can only be valuable if they build on sufficient data and on accurate source materials. To achieve this, it is crucial that a diagnostician ensure a good rendition of discussions and meetings by means of *clinical notes*. In such short, written records is noted down what came up during sessions or what attracted the attention in the functioning of a person. They form the written documentation of clinical meetings and can also include initial hypotheses about the underlying logic recognized in the basic material. Such notes are crucial for the development of subsequent conclusions. Basic psychological research teaches us that as a rule memory is rather biased (Schacter 1999). It would therefore be naïve to expect clinicians to give accurate information about clinical encounters by memory. Clinical notes that are kept during and/or shortly after sessions are far more reliable. On the basis of such notes one can verify whether decisions are well founded in basic clinical material. Supplemented by results from psychological tests, which are sometimes also useful, they represent the material basis of the diagnostic decision-making process.

A classic example of such clinical notes is found with Freud's case study of Ernst Lanzer, a young man who was in therapy with Freud for a few months. What was unique to this case study is that we not only have the published version of it—*Notes Upon A Case of Obsessional Neurosis* (Freud 1909), in which the patient, consistent with his central obsession, is referred to as "the rat man," but also have a part of the clinical working notes that lay at the basis of the case study (Freud 1955). Freud had the habit of destroying such notes as soon as a case was published, which is in line with the deontology of confidentiality that is mandatory in clinical work. The notes about the first and third parts of the treatment of Ernst Lanzer constitute an exception to this rule for reasons that are unclear. Freud (1909, p. 159) reports himself that he wrote these notes "on the evening of the day of treatment, and adhere as closely as possible to my recollection of the patient's words." Paraphrasing literal statements by the patient is interspersed with a report of what was said during the sessions and with comments on how the patient responded non-verbally. Central to these notes is the reproduction of the content of the session. On a secondary level there are also reflections about the underlying dynamic of the case. Nowadays, clinical notes often still exist in a written form. However, in settings where several clinicians work together around one and the same case it might be relevant to work with data processing software for the management of clinical notes. This not only has the advantage of being more easily accessible for authorized colleagues, but also allows clinicians to keep track of indicators to monitor a case, which makes the clinical diagnostic work more transparent vis-a-vis third parties.

In order to stimulate the process of verification and of the cyclic study of clinical notes, and thus to build an authentic work culture around it, peer review and consultation are essential. In mental health care facilities team meetings can be organized around the project of case construction, and starting from their clinical notes clinicians can be charged with formulating hypotheses and conclusions about dynamics and mechanisms that stand out in the materials. Also supervision, work discussion groups, and clinical cartels are primarily intended to stimulate reflection about cases and to get hold of the logic in someone's suffering more accurately. Clinical notes can once again form the basis for such discussions. In terms of giving shape to the verification process colleagues, supervisors and *plus uns* should especially pay attention to the question of *how* and *to what extent* diagnostic statements are well founded in specific clinical material, working notes, and the results of psychological tests, if such tests were deemed relevant. Clinicians would do well to also integrate ideas and concerns arising from team consultation or peer discussions into their work. In this way, these forms of consultation do not result in non-committal freewheeling but provide an impetus to bring order to the notes about a case.

An important point that we retain from the work of Morse et al. (2002) is that ensuring reliability and validity particularly comes down to cultivating a *work culture* in which the decisions made, and the cyclical discussion of basic data, are considered central. In order to achieve this, professional work should be organized such that the process of careful verification is part of regular clinical practice. By integrating the use of clinical notes and work discussion practices into clinical practice, concrete methods to guide the process of ensuring validity and reliability can be established.

However, in qualitative research literature many directives can also be found about the way in which reliability and validity can be established. In line with Morse et al. (2002), these should not so much be used as criteria to check research results, but as principles that might help elaborate the research process in a thoughtful way. In the following sections we focus on how qualitative researchers consider reliability and validity in detail. Once again, we will explore what this implies for the work of clinical diagnosis by means of case formulations.

Reliability Considered Closely

In quantitative research reliability is often seen as an inherent characteristic of a diagnostic tool. In qualitative research, by contrast, reliability is mainly a procedural quality that refers to methodological rigor and transparency (Golafshani 2003). It is a twofold construct that relates to both the quality of the data collected and to the nature of the decision-making process. Hereby, particular attention is paid to the unbiased nature and to the logical consistency of the data collection and analysis.

On the one hand, qualitative research is considered reliable to the extent that it is *unbiased* and one can guarantee that the distortions by the person of the researcher and her context were kept at bay (Lincoln and Guba 1985; Miles and Huberman 1994; Stiles 1993). Conclusions should strongly build on participants' input, and not on the idiosyncrasies of the researcher. In terms of distortion, the literature refers to two major sources of bias. On the one hand, a researcher might be influenced too strongly by personal preconceptions. On the other hand the researcher might sympathize too strongly with the participant, or respond negatively to what she discovers, and as a result, cannot reflect on the data objectively. To control for such bias reflexivity is crucial (Malterud 2001). Reflexivity makes researchers aware of sources of bias.

Very often qualitative researchers include specific control strategies in order to monitor such bias. As such, Miles and Huberman (1994) call on researchers to always *document* what steps they take in the research process. To this end they keep track of considerations and decisions in written form, which can be reviewed during the research process. By writing about the different steps that one takes in the study, reasoning processes are made transparent and verifiable. By means of such documents the researcher can determine whether the conclusions she draws are relevant, and outsiders can also make use of it to check the reasoning steps of the researcher (Lincoln and Guba 1985).

The latter can take shape through consultation and discussion between fellow researchers or via so-called *research audits* (Miles and Huberman 1994). In the event of a research audit a third party verifies and controls whether the conclusions adequately build on the data and do not contain distortions. Such audits should bring researchers to the point of only drawing conclusions that can effectively be confirmed by the data.

Another method of avoiding distortion by the researcher is *triangulation*. Triangulation means that in the generation of findings, one involves different perspectives. This can be done by using various research methods for the collection of data, such as interviews and participatory observation (methodological triangulation). It is also possible to triangulate by involving various researchers in the collection and analysis of the data (triangulation on researchers). Such triangulation does not so much aim at achieving consensus, but at generating a broad perspective of the problem examined. One can also further triangulate by basing the conclusions on several sources (source triangulation). As such one can opt to explicitly study data that are collected at different times or which involve several informants in a study (e.g., the perspective of children as well as of both parents). Triangulation has the primary objective of ensuring well-drafted and well-founded conclusions (Miles and Huberman 1994).

Next to that, reliability also relates to being *logically consistent* in drawing conclusions. Findings must be clearly formulated and justified, and conclusions should be built on facts and premises that are well clarified (Lincoln and Guba 1985). Qualitative researchers monitor this by elucidating their own opinions and by testing provisional conclusions against the judgment of colleagues. Whether conclusions are built consistently and coherently is often examined by research audits, whereby the auditor examines whether the researcher got trapped in fallacies during the research process (ranging from data collection to the documentation of conclusions) (Miles and Huberman 1994). Through such an audit one can check whether each step in the reasoning is sufficiently logically consistent with the previous steps. To make such peer review and verification by external auditors possible, it is of course crucial that the researchers have documented the steps of their research clearly, and keep their material transparently available.

When applied to function-oriented diagnoses by means of case constructions, obtaining good reliability requires that attention is paid to the logical consistency of the clinical decision-making process and to potential sources of bias. This can only be verified if written notes about clinical meetings are available, and if clinicians keep track of how they come to draw conclusions from the basic material. Good clinical notes with reflections on the dynamics in a case and with notes from consultations with third parties are therefore crucial. Such clinical notes enable the clinician to determine whether her decisions are not distorted and were constructed in a logically coherent way. They can also form the basis for a self-critical dialog with third parties in the course of supervision, work discussions, or cartels. Such a dialog can ensure triangulation in the interpretation of clinical material. In view of the risk of flawed thinking and logical reasoning errors in the diagnostic decision-making process (Croskerry 2003; Meehl 1973; Tait 2009), it is of primary importance that special attention is paid to the arguments and reasoning process of a diagnostician. Just like the research auditor, the person in charge of monitoring the process, like the supervisor or the *plus un,* should pay special attention to distortions, incoherencies, or fallacies in the clinician's line of reasoning. Triangulation might also be implemented in the diagnostic context by using different methods for data collection (e.g., discussions, observations, and standardized psychological tests) (= methodical triangulation) and by engaging different informants (source triangulation) in the diagnostic process (e.g., in mapping the perspectives of the child, parents, and teachers with respect to an aggression issue in the child).

A Closer Look at Validity

In qualitative research, validity pertains to the actual correctness and usability of research findings. Often a distinction is made between internal validity or credibility on the one hand, and external validity or transferability on the other hand (Lincoln and Guba 1985; Miles and Huberman 1994).

Internal validity or credibility concerns the correctness of conclusions made and involves the question as to whether the researcher's statements can be accepted as accurate or not. In this context, qualitative researchers usually distance themselves from a realistic epistemology, which assumes that the question as to whether conclusions are true is a matter of correspondence: something is true when it corresponds to objective observations in reality and not true when it is not in accordance with it (Kvale 1995). Qualitative researchers, rather, start off with the assumption that the reality that we experience is largely a socio-culturally determined construction that we actively build. The research that they conduct themselves does not escape this logic, and is therefore also to be regarded as a construction. Questions with respect to the validity of such a scientific construction is not tantamount to checking whether the findings of a researcher are really true, but to verifying in a falsifying way if the conclusions taken are justifiable in the light of the raw research data. Research results are valid when we can reasonably assume that the conclusions taken are *consistently* built on the basic material and give an accurate picture of the actions that respondents take and of the stories they tell. Another criterion to weigh up internal validity concerns the *pragmatic value* of research findings. Within this reasoning conclusions are considered good when they are meaningful, shed an interesting light on the examined phenomenon, and can be used to act in a different and better way in relation to the examined phenomenon (Kvale 1995). Furthermore, conclusions are to be considered as credible when they are sufficiently *nuanced* and indicate what they can or cannot explain in the data (Miles and Huberman 1994). To examine the credibility of research findings, five aspects mentioned below usually pass in review (Lincoln and Guba 1985).

Firstly, qualitative researchers usually appraise how well the researcher is familiarized with the research population. Long-term and intense contact, where one has sufficient time to learn different sides of the examined phenomenon and develop a good personal relationship with participants, is usually considered to be an indicator of good credibility: "If prolonged engagement provides scope, persistent observation provides depth" (Lincoln and Guba 1985, p. 304).

Secondly, triangulation is sometimes regarded as a way to guarantee validity. In terms of validity it is then specifically examined whether or not information from different sources points in the same direction (Miles and Huberman 1994).

A third way to sustain the credibility of research findings is through discussions with colleagues. Lincoln and Guba (1985, p. 308) call this *peer debriefing*. This is done on the basis of the data in dialog with a colleague who is familiar with the field of research, but who is not directly involved in the project. Through such a peer review process, researchers discuss the aspects of consistency, pragmatic usability, and nuance, which we have just indicated. The underlying idea is that peers may be critical dialog partners, and that their opinion constitutes an interesting standard to which the plausibility of decisions can be assessed. Concretely, such peer debriefing can be included in a research audit, which thus has an eye not only for the reliability of the research work, but also for the validity of the findings.

A fourth strategy to enhance the credibility of a qualitative research project is by addressing and discussing *negative cases* or material that does not fit within the picture the researcher constructs. By exploring enough material that contradicts the overall results, a researcher is encouraged to clarify her findings. This also allows for a realistic framing of the conclusions (Lincoln and Guba 1985).

A fifth way to underpin the credibility of research findings is by bringing these into *dialog* with theories and research results from earlier studies (Miles and Huberman 1994). Crucial to this is not so much *whether* the findings confirm earlier work and insights, but *how* new results can be viewed in light of other work and theories, and vice versa. Credible research findings specify how and to what extent a theory is applicable to the collected data and stipulate how the conclusions of the studies carried out are connected with results from similar research.

External validity or transferability refers to the extent to which the findings from a specific study can be generalized and apply to other cases and other contexts. Lincoln and Guba (1985) stress that such a generalization is only possible if the researchers sufficiently detail, contextualize, and document their findings. Only when such details are given can other researchers examine to what extent findings on other situations, persons, times, and *settings* are applicable to their contexts. Lincoln and Guba (1985) talk in this context about the need for *thick descriptions*. This means that researchers have to provide sufficient details concerning who the participants are, under what conditions and with what intensity the data was collected, and in which social-cultural context the study is happening. For case studies, such detail is crucial. Transferability of one case to another is only possible when crucial characteristics are described in sufficient detail. Furthermore, information pertaining to whether findings could be *replicated* or not contribute to the external validity of a study. Conversely, statements about the extent to which a study confirms or complements the results of previous research are also relevant at this level.

These principles concerning credibility and transferability are also pertinent in the light of clinical case construction and encourage devoting attention to the validity of the clinical decision-making process in function-oriented diagnosis. A number of the specific procedures that we have already outlined in the sections about reflexivity and reliability are relevant on this point, provided that they also concentrate on aspects of validity.

In order to be able to guarantee good internal validity, clinicians should first of all ensure that case formulations are well attuned to the clinical data gathered during diagnostic sessions (discussions, observations, psychological testing). In times of *efficiency*, pressure can be exercised to limit the number of diagnostic sessions with patients. Considered from the perspective of validity such pressure is not beneficial. To truly assess someone's problems in detail, and to do justice to the complexity of a person's experiences and functioning, sufficient clinical contact is indispensable. Only by spending sufficient time on the diagnostic assessment can one prepare well-founded interventions. Furthermore, clinical notes in which meetings with the patient are carefully documented are also crucial. The internal validity of a case construction is stronger when there is clear evidence that a diagnostician is very *familiar* with the basic material. Furthermore, *triangulation* is also important. Where possible, clinical data are best collected by using different methods (e.g., open interviews and observations), informants (e.g., a child and his parents), and/or clinicians (e.g., psychologist and departmental nurse). If triangulation brings out similar points in a consistent manner, one can be more confident that these facets are really important within a person's functioning. Triangulation doesn't, however, always deliver converging viewpoints, and the basic material that one maps via clinical notes often also contains inconsistencies and anomalies. By paying explicit attention to inconsistent information the validity of the case formulation increases. Contradictory evidence allows one to nuance conclusions and to estimate the relative value of inferences from the data. Furthermore, one can also underpin the internal validity of a case construction by explicitly bringing the logic that one observes in a case into *dialog* with *theoretical lines of reasoning, other case studies, or research findings.* Herewith it is of course important not to reason paradigmatically and not to cram the case into the straitjacket of established ideas. Theories, other case studies, and research findings are useful when they act as a compass and draw the diagnostician's attention to remarkable patterns in the case material. Instead of applying theories to a case, one should apply the case to theories. Elements that are surprising in the light of the existing corpus of knowledge often strongly reflect the singularities of the case. Validation does not imply that the diagnostician merely "proves" that a case is consistent with the literature, but that she makes the effort of illuminating the specificity of the case in the light of existing knowledge.

A last strategy that qualitative researchers apply to optimize the internal validity of their studies is *peer debriefing*. In clinical contexts this implies that diagnosticians do well to subject their decision-making process to peer review. Supervision, work discussions, or clinical cartels offer an interesting forum to speak with colleagues about how well diagnostic conclusions are rooted in the clinical material. Meehl (1973) has noted that clinicians often draw far-reaching conclusions about patients on the basis of staggeringly little material. One can go against this tendency toward hasty decision-making by paying explicit attention to the soundness of clinical conclusions. By drawing on the critical inquiry of peers the internal validity of a case formulation increases.

In addition to internal validity, the question of transferability or external validity is also high on the agenda of the qualitative researcher. What is important in this context is the need to develop thick descriptions. Applied to function-oriented diagnosis this means that case formulations should be sufficiently detailed, and that decisions about the functioning of a person must be properly contextualized. *Providing detail* in the diagnosis is extremely important in terms of developing good interventions and enhancing the accuracy of discussions with peers. In order to build an accurate idea, it is important that all relevant information is reported clearly and with sufficient detail. When, in a subsequent step, the patient is referred to a colleague, the same applies. In order to avoid repetition of the whole diagnostic process, the logic observed in the case needs to be communicated properly. Clear and well-documented clinical reports are essential for this. In addition, paying sufficient attention to contextualization warrants external validity. This implies that the diagnostician clearly reports on how the patient's functioning is embedded in specific life contexts, and also shows the circumstances under which the diagnostic process itself took place. Only by clarifying the diagnostic context can diagnostic findings be transferred in a valid way. Regarding generalization across cases, it is advisable to always be careful and to do justice to the singularity of a case. In line with our concerns formulated in Chap. 3 it is important to have an eye both for peculiarities and for singularities in someone's functioning. Often diagnosticians are able to distinguish particular dynamics in someone's functioning that are in line with our existing knowledge. Obviously such particularities should be described well in a case formulation. In addition, however, singularities need to be clearly discussed and documented as well.

Conclusion

In this chapter we focused on function-oriented diagnosis, suggesting that case formulations constitute a viable alternative for classificatory DSM diagnosis. Function-oriented diagnosis does not aim at classification, but maps how problems and symptoms are embedded in someone's wider functioning. Case formulations can be constructed on the basis of concrete material from clinical meetings, observation data, and information from psychological testing. The diagnostician discusses this material with the aim of making clear *how* problems are organized. The net result of function-oriented diagnosis is a narrative formulation that highlights the specificities of someone's problems and strengths, which also indicates how a person's functioning is embedded in relevant contexts.

In our discussion of the DSM we were very critical of the scientific status of this prestigious psychiatric diagnostic manual. We deemed its reliability and validity as insufficient. Is function-oriented diagnosis on this point so much more robust? The discussion around reflexivity, reliability, and validity in this chapter will have made it clear that this is not automatically the case. In diagnostic measurement tools arising from a positivistic research approach, reliability and validity are properties that appear to be inherent to the instrument itself. In large-scale studies researchers investigate how an instrument scores on a series of quality indicators, and on condition that users adhere to the testing protocol, one accepts that the findings of the large-scale study also apply to individual diagnostic situations. Case formulations, by contrast, are reasoned narrative constructions that do not simply fit within this research tradition. To assess the quality of case constructions we can appeal to methodological literature on qualitative research. This literature suggests that researchers need to work reflexively and give shape to the reliability and validity of their research through various methods. In this chapter I therefore propose that the diagnostician who works with case formulations should monitor and enhance the quality of her narratively based work, similar to the qualitative researcher. Function-oriented diagnosis requires a quality policy in which the reflexivity, reliability, and validity of the diagnostic process are established as well as possible. The principles and methods presented in this chapter may be used as a guide in this context.

Some readers may get the impression that with our plea for function-oriented diagnoses we are taking a step backward in time, since the common language of the DSM is no longer useful. For example, anyone working with the DSM knows the core diagnostic features of a serious depression. Is there no risk that abandoning the DSM will lead to confusion since a shared terminology to assess different kinds of psychopathology is therefore removed? This risk does exist but it is not insurmountable. On the one hand, the reassurance obtained through the common language of the DSM is largely an illusion. What is a shared language worth if the users of it give substantially different interpretations of the terminology with which it is made up? The poor results from the DSM-5 reliability studies show that there is little consistency in how diagnosticians handle the DSM. On the other hand, it is important that clinicians can clearly communicate with each other. To achieve this, psy-professionals need to pay more attention to the development of *a common language around symptoms of psychopathology*. In the DSM one hardly finds definitions or descriptions which make it clear, for example, what a hallucination exactly is and how it differs from a perceptual illusion, or what the core features of problematic forgetfulness in school children are. The DSM focuses too much on distinguishing syndromes. In the future we must pay more attention to the elaboration of a descriptive catalogue of symptoms.

Furthermore, our plea for function-oriented diagnosis can give the impression that we think of syndromes in a very relativistic way. Are all cases so unique that generalization is hardly possible? I do not think so. In line with Van Os (2013) or following Lacan's differentiation between clinical structures (see Chap. 3), I believe that it is useful to distinguish groups of problems within the broad field of psychopathology. For example, it makes sense to differentiate between psychoses and neurotic conditions, and to discern addictions from neurocognitive disorders. When accepting broad groupings on the basis of typical core symptoms, we maintain a global picture of kinds of psychopathology, but immediately also bring into account that case-specific singularities are crucial.

Finally, our plea for function-oriented diagnosis might create uncertainty in terms of the differential diagnostic distinction between pathological and non-pathological functioning. Will function-oriented diagnostics not result in all functioning being problematized? I think that the reverse is true. In fact, the DSM is in danger of psychiatrizing behavior from which people do not seriously suffer (see Chap. 4). Case formulation enables a contextualized discussion of symptoms and painful issues in people's lives, as well as strengths that add to their resilience. This is crucial in terms of establishing personalized interventions in mental health care.

Other References

Balint, M. (1957). *The doctor, his patient and the illness*. London: Pitman Medical.
Borsboom, D., & Cramer, A. O. J. (2013). Network analysis: An integrative approach to the structure of psychopathology. *Annual Review of Clinical Psychology, 9*, 91–121.
Borsboom, D., Cramer, A. O. J., Schmittmann, V. D., Epskamp, S., & Waldorp, L. J. (2011). The small world of psychopathology. *PLoS ONE, 6*, e27407.
Bradley, J. (2008). The work discussion seminar: A learning environment. In M. Rustin & J. Bradley (Eds.), *Work discussion* (pp. 22–37). London: Karnac.
Bruner, J. (1990). *Acts of meaning*. Cambridge: Harvard University Press.
Bruner, J. (1991). The narrative construction of reality. *Critical Inquiry, 18*, 1–21.
Croskerry, P. (2003). The importance of cognitive errors in diagnosis and strategies to minimize them. *Academic Medicine, 78*, 775–780.
de La Mettrie, J.O. (1747). L'homme machine. Retrieved July 21, 2014, from http://fr.wikisource.org/wiki/L%27Homme_Machine.
Faber, B. A., Brink, D. C., & Raskin, P. M. (1996). *The psychotherapy of Carl Rogers: Cases and commentary*. New York: Guilford.
Farnan, J. M., Petty, L. A., Georgitis, E., Martin, S., Chiu, E., Prochaska, M., & Arora, V. M. (2012). A systematic review: The effect of clinical supervision on patient and residency education outcomes. *Academic Medicine, 87*, 428–442.
Ferenczi, S. (1995). *The clinical diary of Sándor Ferenczi*. Cambridge: Harvard University Press.

Fichtner, G. (2010). Freud and the Hammerschlag family: A formative relationship. *International Journal of Psychoanalysis, 91*, 1137–1156.

Foucault, M. (1973–1974). *Psychiatric power – Lectures at the Collège de France.* New York: Picador.

Foucault, M. (2006 [1973–74]). *Psychiatric power – Lectures at the Collège de France.* New York: Picador.

Franklin, C. S., & Ballan, M. (2001). Reliability and validity in qualitative research. In B. A. Thyer (Ed.), *The handbook of social work research methods* (pp. 273–292). Thousand Oaks: Sage.

Freud, S., & Breuer J. (1895). Studies on hysteria. In J. Strachey (Ed. and Trans.), *The standard edition of the complete psychological works of Sigmund Freud* (Vol. 2, pp. 1–335). London: Hogarth Press.

Freud, S. (1953 [1900]). The interpretation of dreams. In *The standard edition of the complete psychological works for Sigmund Freud* (Vols. 4, 5). London: Hogarth Press.

Freud, S. (1953 [1901]). The psychopathology of everyday life. In *The standard edition of the complete psychological works for Sigmund Freud* (Vol. 6). London: Hogarth Press.

Freud, S. (1953 [1905a]). The jokes and their relation to the unconscious. In *The standard edition of the complete psychological works for Sigmund Freud* (Vol. 8). London: Hogarth Press.

Freud, S. (1953 [1905b]). Fragments of an analysis of a case of hysteria. In *The standard edition of the complete psychological works for Sigmund Freud* (Vol. 7, pp. 1–122). London: Hogarth Press.

Freud, S. (1953 [1909]). Notes upon a case of obsessional neurosis. In *The standard edition of the complete psychological works for Sigmund Freud* (Vol. 10, pp. 153–318). London: Hogarth Press.

Freud, S. (1955). Notes upon a case of obsessional neurosis (The Rat Man) (Part I). In J. Strachey (Ed. and Trans.), *The standard edition of the complete psychological works of Sigmund Freud* (Vol. 10, pp. 158–220). London: Hogarth Press.

Golafshani, N. (2003). Understanding reliability and validity in qualitative research. *The qualitative Report, 8*, 597–607.

Harper, D. (2012). Online etymological dictionary. Retrieved via: http://www.etymonline.com

Hendriksen, J. (2009). *Handboek Intervisie [Intervision manual].* Barneveld: Nelissen.

Highet, N., Stevenson, A. L., Purtell, C., & Coo, S. (2014). Qualitative insights into women's personal experiences of perinatal depression and anxiety. *Women and Birth, 27*, 179–184.

Kanfer, F. H., & Saslow, G. (1965). Behavioral analysis – An alternative to diagnostic classification. *Archives of General Psychiaty, 12*, 529–538.

Kvale, S. (1995). The social construction of validity. *Qualitative Inquiry, 1*, 19–40.

Lacan, J. (1964). *The seminar 1964, book XI, the four fundamental concepts of psycho-analysis*. London/New York: Karnac.

Lacan, J. (1975). Conférences et entretiens dans des universités nord-americaines [Conferences and interviews at North-American universities]. *Scilicet, 6/7*, 42–45.

Lacan, J. (2006 [1956a]). The situation of psychoanalysis and the training of psychoanalysts in 1956. In J. Lacan & J. A. Miller (Eds.), *Écrits* (pp. 384–411). New York/London: W. W. Norton.

Lacan, J. (1956b). Discours de Rome [The Rome discourse]. In J. Lacan (Ed.), *Autres Écrits* (pp. 133–165). Paris: Seuil.

Lacan, J. (2006 [1959]). On a question prior to any possible treatment of psychosis. In J. Lacan & J. A. Miller (Eds.), *Écrits* (pp. 445–488). New York/London: W. W. Norton.

Lacan, J. (2006 [1961]). The direction of treatment and the principles of its power. In J. Lacan & J. A. Miller (Eds.), *Écrits* (pp. 489–542). New York/London: W. W. Norton.

Lévi-Strauss, C. (1958). *Antropologie structurale [Structural antrophology]*. Paris: Plon.

Lemaire, T. (2008). *Claude Lévi-Strauss. Tussen mythe en muziek [Claude Lévi-Strauss. In between myth and music]*. Amsterdam: Ambo.

Lincoln, Y. S., & Guba, E. G. (1985). *Naturalistic inquiry*. Newbury Park: Sage.

Madill, A., & Gough, B. (2008). Qualitative research and its place in psychological science. *Psychological Methods, 13*, 254–271.

Malterud, K. (2001). Qualitative research: Standards, challenges, and guidelines. *The Lancet, 358*, 483–488.

Marecek, J. (2003). Dancing through minefields: Towards a qualitative stance in psychology. In P. M. Camic, J. E. Rhodes, & L. Yardley (Eds.), *Qualtitative research in psychology* (pp. 49–69). Washington, DC: American Psychological Association.

Marková, I. S., & Berrios, G. E. (2009). Epistemology of mental symptoms. *Psychopathology, 42*, 343–349.

Meehl, P. E. (1973). Why I do not attend case conferences. In *Psychodiagnosis: Selected papers* (pp. 225–302). Minneapolis: University of Minnesota Press.

Merleau-Ponty, M. (1945). *La Phénoménologie de la Perception [The phenomenology of perception]*. Paris: Gallimard.

Miles, M., & Huberman, M. (1994). *Qualitative data analysis*. London: Sage.

Miller, J. A. (1983). Pas de Clinique sans éthique [No clinic without ethics]. *Actes de l'ECF, 5*, 65–68.

Miller, S., Hubble, M., & Duncan, B. (2007). Supershrinks – What's the secret of their success? *Psychotherapy Networker, 31*(6).

Mor Barak, M. E., Travis, D. J., Pyun, H., & Xie, B. (2009). The impact of supervision on worker outcomes: A meta-analysis. *The Social Service Review, 83*(1), 3–32.

Morse, J. M., Barrett, M., Mayan, M., Olson, K., & Spiers, J. (2002). Verification strategies for establishing reliability and validity in qualitative research. *International Journal of Qualitative Methods, 1*(2), Article 2.

Parker, I. (2005). *Qualitative psychology: Introducing radical research*. Maidenhead/New York: Open University Press.

Polkinghorne, D. (1990). Language and qualitative research. *Theoretical and Philosophical Psychology, 10*, 3–24.

Ponterotto, J. G. (2005). Qualitative research in counselling psychology: A primer on research paradigms and philosophy of science. *Journal of Counseling Psychology, 52*, 126–136.

Richardson, L. (1994). Writing: A method of inquiry. In N. K. Denzin & Y. S. Lincoln (Eds.), *Handbook of qualitative research* (pp. 516–529). Thousand Oaks: Sage.

Schacter, D. L. (1999). The seven sins of memory: Insights from psychology and cognitive neuroscience. *American Psychologist, 54*, 182–203.

Showalter, E. (1998). *Hystories*. New York: Columbia University Press.

Stiles, W. B. (1993). Quality control in qualitative research. *Clinical Psychology Review, 13*, 593–618.

Sturmey, P. (2009). Case formulation: A review and overview of this volume. In P. Sturmey (Ed.), *Clinical case formulation: Varieties of approaches* (pp. 3–32). Oxford: Wiley-Blackwell.

Tait, G. (2009). The logic of ADHD: A brief review of fallacious reasoning. *Studies in Philosophy and Education, 28*, 239–254.

Temerlin, M. K. (1968). Suggestion effects in psychiatric diagnosis. *Journal of Nervous and Mental Disease, 147*, 349–353.

Temerlin, M. K. (1970). Diagnostic bias in community mental health. *Community Mental Health Journal, 6*, 110–117.

Van Os, J. (2010). Are psychiatric diagnoses of psychosis scientific and useful? The case of schizophrenia. *Journal of Mental Health, 19*, 305–317.

Van Os, J. (2013). *De DSM-5 voorbij! [Beyond DSM-5!]*. Leusden: Diagnosis uitgevers.

Van Roy, K., Vanheule, S., Debaere, V., Inslegers, R., Meganck, R., & Deganck, J. (2014). A Lacanian view on Balint group meetings: A qualitative analysis of two case presentations. *BMC Family Practice, 15*, 49. doi:10.1186/1471-2296-15-49.

Vanheule, S., & Verhaeghe, P. (2004). Powerlessness and impossibility in special education: A qualitative study on professional burnout from a Lacanian perspective. *Human Relations, 57*, 497–519.

Vanheule, S., Lievrouw, A., & Verhaeghe, P. (2003). Burnout and intersubjectivity: A psychoanalytical study from a Lacanian perspective. *Human Relations, 56*, 321–339.

Verhaeghe, P. (2002). *On being normal and other disorders*. New York: Other Press.

Watt, D. (2007). On becoming a qualitative researcher: The value of reflexivity. *The Qualitative Report, 12*, 82–101.

Wigman, J. T. W., van Os, J., Thiery, E., et al. (2013). Psychiatric diagnosis revisited: Towards a system of staging and profiling combining nomothetic and idiographic parameters of momentary mental states. *PLoS ONE, 8*, e59559.

Wundt, W. (1897). *Outlines of psychology*. Leipzig: Wilhelm Engelman.

Bibliography

Throughout the book, references to subsequent versions of the DSM used the following abbreviations: DSM-I, DSM-II, DSM-III, DSM-III-R, DSM-IV, DSM-IV-TR, DSM-5. These are the complete references to these manuals:

American Psychiatric Association. (1952). *Diagnostic and statistical manual of mental disorders – Second edition – DSM-I*. Washington, DC: American Psychiatric Association.
American Psychiatric Association. (1968). *Diagnostic and statistical manual of mental disorders – Second edition – DSM-II*. Washington, DC: American Psychiatric Association.
American Psychiatric Association. (1980). *Diagnostic and statistical manual of mental disorders – Third edition – DSM-III*. Washington, DC: American Psychiatric Association.
American Psychiatric Association. (1994). *Diagnostic and statistical manual of mental disorders – Fourth edition – DSM-IV*. Washington, DC: American Psychiatric Association.
American Psychiatric Association. (2000). *Diagnostic and statistical manual of mental disorders – Fourth edition, text revision – DSM-IV-TR*. Washington, DC: American Psychiatric Association.

American Psychiatric Association. (2013). *Diagnostic and statistical manual of mental disorders – Fifth edition – DSM-5*. Washington, DC: American Psychiatric Association.

Other References

Adriaens, P., & De Block, A. (2013). Why we essentialize mental disorders. *Journal of Medicine and Philosophy, 38*, 107–127.

American Medico-Psychological Association & National Committee for Mental Hygiene. (1918). *Statistical manual for the use of institutions for the insane*. New York: National Committee for Mental Hygiene. Retrieved October 2, 2013, from http://archive.org/stream/statisticalmanu00assogoog#page/n32/mode/2up.

Andreasen, N. (2001). Diversity in psychiatry: Or, why did we become psychiatrists? *American Journal of Psychiatry, 158*, 673–675.

Angermeyer, M. C., Holzinger, A., Carta, M. G., & Schomerus, G. (2011). Biogenetic explanations and public acceptance of mental illness: Systematic review of population studies. *The British Journal of Psychiatry, 199*, 367–372.

Angst, J. (2002). Historical aspects of the dichotomy between manic-depressive disorders and schizophrenia. *Schizophrenia Research, 57*, 5–13.

Baer, L., & Blais, M. A. (2010). *Handbook of clinical rating scales and assessment in psychiatry and mental health*. New York: Humana Press.

Balint, M. (1957). *The doctor, his patient and the illness*. London: Pitman Medical.

Barone, D. F., et al. (2005). Increasing empathic accuracy through practice and feedback in clinical interviewing course. *Journal of Social and Clinical Psychology, 24*, 156–171.

Batstra, L., & Thoutenhoofd, E. D. (2012). The risk that DSM-5 will further inflate the diagnostic bubble. *Current Psychiatry Reviews, 8*, 260–263.

Beavan, V., Read, J., & Cartwright, C. (2011). The prevalence of voice-hearers in the general population: A literature review. *Journal of Mental Health, 20*, 281–292.

Beck, A. T., Ward, C. H., Mendelson, M., Mock, J. E., & Erbaugh, J. K. (1962). Reliability of psychiatric diagnoses: 2. A study of consistency of clinical judgments and ratings. *American Journal of Psychiatry, 119*, 351–357.

Ben-Zeev, D., Young, M. A., & Corrigan, P. W. (2010). DSM-V and the stigma of mental illness. *Journal of Mental Health, 19*, 318–327.

Bergmann, J. R. (1992). Veiled morality: Notes on discretion in psychiatry. In P. Drew & J. Heritage (Eds.), *Talk at work: Interaction in institutional settings* (pp. 137–162). Cambridge: Cambridge University Press.

Bernstein, C. A. (2011). Meta-structure in DSM-5 process. *Psychiatric News, 46*(5), 7–29.

Berrios, G. E. (1992). Phenomenology, psychopathology and Jaspers: A conceptual history. *History of Psychiatry, 3*, 303–327.

Berrios, G. E. (1999). Classifications in psychiatry: A conceptual history. *Australian and New Zealand Journal of Psychiatry, 33*, 145–160.

Berrios, G. E. (2012). The 19th-century nosology of alienism: History and epistemology. In K. S. Kendler & J. Parnas (Eds.), *Philosophical issues in psychiatry II – Nosology* (pp. 101–117). Oxford: Oxford University Press.

Berrios, G. E., & Hauser, R. (1988). The early development of Kraepelin's ideas on classification: A conceptual history. *Psychological Medicine, 18*, 813–821.

Berrios, G. E., & Marková, I. S. (2002). Conceptual issues. In H. D'haenen, J. A. den Boer, & P. Willner (Eds.), *Biological psychiatry* (pp. 9–39). Chichester: Wiley.

Berrios, G. E., & Marková, I. S. (2006). Symptoms: Historical perspective and effect on diagnosis. In M. Blumenfield & J. J. Strain (Eds.), *Psychosomatic medicine* (pp. 27–38). Philadelphia: Lippincott Williams & Wilkins.

Bird, A., & Tobin, E. (2010). Natural kinds. In E. N. Zalta (Ed.), *The Stanford encyclopedia of philosophy (Summer 2010 edition)*. Retrieved September 16, 2011, from http://plato.stanford.edu/archives/sum2010/entries/natural-kinds/.

Blatt, S. J., & Zuroff, D. C. (2005). Empirical evaluation of the assumptions in identifying evidence based treatments in mental health. *Clinical Psychology Review, 25*, 459–486.

Bleuler, E. (1934). *Textbook of psychiatry*. New York: Macmillan.

Bolton, D. (2013). Overdiagnosis problems in the DSM-IV and the new DSM-5: Can they be resolved by the distress – Impairment criterion? *Canadian Journal of Psychiatry, 58*, 612–617.

Borsboom, D., & Cramer, A. O. J. (2013). Network analysis: An integrative approach to the structure of psychopathology. *Annual Review of Clinical Psychology, 9*, 91–121.

Borsboom, D., Cramer, A. O. J., Schmittmann, V. D., Epskamp, S., & Waldorp, L. J. (2011). The small world of psychopathology. *PLoS ONE, 6*, e27407.

Boschloo, L., van Borkulo, C. D., Rhemtulla, M., Keyes, K. M., Borsboom, D., & Schoevers, R. A. (2015). The network structure of symptoms of the diagnostic and statistical manual of mental disorders. *PLoS ONE, 10*, e0137621.

Bracken, P., Thomas, P., Timimi, S., et al. (2012). Psychiatry beyond the current paradigm. *British Journal of Psychiatry, 201*, 430–434.
Bradley, J. (2008). The work discussion seminar: A learning environment. In M. Rustin & J. Bradley (Eds.), *Work discussion* (pp. 22–37). London: Karnac.
Bruner, J. (1990). *Acts of meaning*. Cambridge: Harvard University Press.
Bruner, J. (1991). The narrative construction of reality. *Critical Inquiry, 18*, 1–21.
Buchheim, A., Viviani, R., Kessler, H., et al. (2013). Changes in prefrontal-limbic function in major depression after 15 months of long-term psychotherapy. *Plos One, 7*, e33745.
Canguilhem, G. (1966). *The normal and the pathological*. Brooklyn: Zone Books.
Carey, B. (2008, December 17). Psychiatrists revise the book of human troubles. *New York Times*.
Charney, D. S., Barlow, D. H., Botteron, K., et al. (2002). Neuroscience research agenda to guide development of a pathophysiologically based classification system. In D. J. Kupfer, M. B. First, & D. A. Regier (Eds.), *A research agenda for DSM-V* (pp. 31–83). Washington, DC: American Psychiatric Association.
Chmielewski, M., Bagby, R. M., Clark, L. A., & Watson, D. (2015). Method matters: Understanding diagnostic reliability in DSM-IV and DSM-5. *Journal of Abnormal Psychology, 124*, 764–769.
Clarke, D. E., Narrow, W. E., Regier, D. A., et al. (2013). DSM-5 field trials in the United States and Canada, part I: Study design, sampling strategy, implementation, and analytic approaches. *American Journal of Psychiatry, 170*, 43–58.
Compton, W. M., & Guze, S. B. (1995). The neo-Kraepelinian revolution in psychiatric diagnosis. *European Archives of Psychiatry and Clinical Neuroscience, 245*, 196–201.
Cooper, R. (2005). *Classifying madness – A philosophical examination of the diagnostic and statistical manual of mental disorders*. Dordrecht: Springer.
Cooper, R. (2007). *Psychiatry and philosophy of science*. Stocksfield: Acumen.
Cosgrove, L., & Krimsky, S. (2012). A comparison of DSM-IV and DSM-5 panel members' financial associations with industry: A pernicious problem persists. *Plos Medicine, 9*, e1001190.
Cosgrove, L., Krimsky, S., Vijayaraghavan, M., & Schneider, L. (2006). Financial ties between DSM-IV panel members and the pharmaceutical industry. *Psychotherapy and Psychosomatics, 75*, 154–180.
Cosgrove, L., Krimsky, S., Wheeler, E. E., et al. (2014). Tripartite conflicts of interest and high stakes patent extensions in the DSM-5. *Psychotherapy and Psychosomatics, 83*, 106–113.

Croskerry, P. (2003). The importance of cognitive errors in diagnosis and strategies to minimize them. *Academic Medicine, 78*, 775–780.

Damasio, A. (2010). *Self comes to mind: Constructing the conscious brain*. New York: Vintage.

Dar-Nimrod, I., & Heine, S. J. (2011). Genetic essentialism: On the deceptive determinism of DNA. *Psychological Bulletin, 137*, 800–818.

de La Mettrie, J.O. (1747). L'homme machine. Retrieved July 21, 2014, from http://fr.wikisource.org/wiki/L%27Homme_Machine.

de Saussure, F. (1916). *Course in general linguistics*. New York: Philosophical Library.

De Vos, J. (2014). Which materialism? Questioning the matrix of psychology, neurology, psychoanalysis and ideology critique. *Theory and Psychology, 24*, 76–92.

Decker, H. (2007). How Kraepelinian was Kraepelin? How Kraepelinian are the neo-Kraepelinians? – from Emil Kraepelin to DSM-III. *History of Psychiatry, 18*, 337–360.

Decker, H. (2013). *The making of DSM-III*. New York: Oxford University Press.

DeFife, J. A., Peart, J., Bradley, B., et al. (2013). Validity of prototype diagnosis for mood and anxiety disorders. *JAMA Psychiatry, 70*, 140–148.

Dehue, T. (2008). *De depressie-epidemie. Over de plicht het lot in eigen hand te nemen [The depression epidemic. On the duty to control your own destiny]*. Amsterdam: Augustus.

Dennett, D. C. (1991). *Consciousness explained*. Boston: Little Brown.

Dowrick, C. (2009). *Beyond depression: A new approach to understanding and management*. Oxford: Oxford University Press.

Dubovsky, S. L. (2016). The limitations of genetic testing in psychiatry. *Psychotherapy and Psychosomatics, 85*, 129–135.

Eco, U. (1976). *A theory of semiotics*. London: Macmillan.

Evrard, R. (2013). Psychopathology and exceptional experiences: A literature review. *L'Évolution Psychiatrique, 78*, 155–176.

Faber, B. A., Brink, D. C., & Raskin, P. M. (1996). *The psychotherapy of Carl Rogers: Cases and commentary*. New York: Guilford.

Farnan, J. M., Petty, L. A., Georgitis, E., Martin, S., Chiu, E., Prochaska, M., & Arora, V. M. (2012). A systematic review: The effect of clinical supervision on patient and residency education outcomes. *Academic Medicine, 87*, 428–442.

Feighner, J. P., Woodruff, R. A., Winokur, G., Munoz, R., Robins, E., & Guze, S. B. (1972). Diagnostic criteria for use in psychiatric research. *Archives of General Psychiatry, 26*, 57–63.

Ferenczi, S. (1995). *The clinical diary of Sándor Ferenczi*. Cambridge: Harvard University Press.

Feyaerts, J., & Vanheule, S. (2015). How to return to subjectivity? Natorp, Husserl and Lacan on the limits of reflection. *Theory & Psychology, 25,* 753–774.

Fichtner, G. (2010). Freud and the Hammerschlag family: A formative relationship. *International Journal of Psychoanalysis, 91,* 1137–1156.

First, M. B., Spitzer, R. L., Gibbon, M., et al. (1995). The structured clinical interview for DSM-III-R personality disorders (SCID-II). Part II: Multi-site test-retest reliability study. *Journal of Personality Disorders, 9,* 92–104.

First, M. B., Williams, J. B. W., Karg, R. S., & Spitzer, R. L. (2016). *Structured clinical interview for DSM-5 disorders – Clinican version (SCID-5-CV).* Washington, DC: American Psychiatric Association.

Fleiss, J. L., & Cohen, J. (1973). The equivalence of weighted kappa and the intraclass correlation coefficient as measures of reliability. *Educational and Psychological Measurement, 33,* 613–619.

Fleiss, J. L., Levin, B., & Paik, M. (1981). The measurement of interrater agreement. In J. L. Fleiss, B. Levin, & M. C. Paik (Eds.), *Statistical methods for rates and proportions – Third edition* (pp. 598–626). New York: Wiley.

Foucault, M. (1965). *Madness and civilization: A history of insanity in the age of reason.* New York: Random House.

Foucault, M. (2006 [1973–74]). *Psychiatric power – Lectures at the Collège de France.* New York: Picador.

Frances, A. (2012, May 8). *Newsflash from APA meeting: DSM-5 has flunked its reliability tests.* Retrieved May 19, 2013, from http://www.huffingtonpost.com/allen-frances/DSM-5-reliability-tests_b_1490857.html.

Frances, A. (2013). *Saving normal – An insider's revolt against out-of-control psychiatric diagnosis, DSM-5, big pharma, and the medicalization of ordinary life.* New York: William Morrow & Harper Collins Publishers.

Franklin, C. S., & Ballan, M. (2001). Reliability and validity in qualitative research. In B. A. Thyer (Ed.), *The handbook of social work research methods* (pp. 273–292). Thousand Oaks: Sage.

Freedman, R., Lewis, D. A., Michels, R., et al. (2013). The initial field trials of DSM-5: New blooms and old thorns. *American Journal of Psychiatry, 170,* 1–5.

Freud, S., & Breuer J. (1895). Studies on hysteria. In J. Strachey (Ed. and Trans.), *The standard edition of the complete psychological works of Sigmund Freud* (Vol. 2, pp. 1–335). London: Hogarth Press.

Freud, S. (1953 [1900]). The interpretation of dreams. In *The standard edition of the complete psychological works for Sigmund Freud* (Vols. 4, 5). London: Hogarth Press.

Freud, S. (1953 [1901]). The psychopathology of everyday life. In *The standard edition of the complete psychological works for Sigmund Freud* (Vol. 6). London: Hogarth Press.

Freud, S. (1953 [1905a]). The jokes and their relation to the unconscious. In *The standard edition of the complete psychological works for Sigmund Freud* (Vol. 8). London: Hogarth Press.

Freud, S. (1953 [1905b]). Fragments of an analysis of a case of hysteria. In *The standard edition of the complete psychological works for Sigmund Freud* (Vol. 7, pp. 1–122). London: Hogarth Press.

Freud, S. (1953 [1909]). Notes upon a case of obsessional neurosis. In *The standard edition of the complete psychological works for Sigmund Freud* (Vol. 10, pp. 153–318). London: Hogarth Press.

Freud, S. (1953 [1913]). On beginning the treatment (Further recommendations on the technique of psychoanalysis I). In *The standard edition of the complete psychological works for Sigmund Freud* (Vol. 12, pp. 121–144). London: Hogarth Press.

Freud, S. (1953 [1917]). Mourning and Melancholia. In *The standard edition of the complete psychological works for Sigmund Freud* (Vol. 14, pp. 243–258). London: Hogarth Press.

Gagnon, M. A., & Lexchin, J. (2008). The cost of pushing pills: A new estimate of pharmaceutical promotion expenditures in the United States. *PLoS Med, 5*(1), e1.

Gandin, T. (2013). *The autistic brain – Thinking across the spectrum.* Boston: Houghton, Mifflin Harcourt.

Gantt, E. E. (2000). Levinas, psychotherapy, and the ethics of suffering. *Journal of Humanistic Psychology, 40,* 9–28.

Golafshani, N. (2003). Understanding reliability and validity in qualitative research. *The qualitative Report, 8,* 597–607.

Good, B. J. (1994). *Medicine, rationality, and experience. An anthropological perspective.* Cambridge: Cambridge University Press.

Grob, G. N. (1987). The forging of mental health policy in America: World War II to new frontier. *Journal of the History of Medicine and Allied Sciences, 42,* 410–446.

Grob, G. N. (1991). Origins of DSM-I: A study in appearance and reality. *American Journal of Psychiatry, 148,* 421–431.

Guze, S. B. (1992). *Why psychiatry is a branch of medicine.* New York: Oxford University Press.

Hacking, I. (2002). Inaugural lecture: Chair of philosophy and history of science concepts at the Collège de France, 16 January 2001. *Economy and Society, 31,* 1–14.

Haggerty, G., Zodan, J., Zubair, A., et al. (2016). Reliability and validity of prototype diagnosis for adolescent psychopathology. *The Journal of Nervous and Mental Disease, 204*, 287–290.

Harper, D. (2011). *Online etymological dictionary*. Retrieved September 7, 2011, from http://www.etymonline.com/index.php?search=diagnosis.

Harwood, V. (2010). Mobile asylums: Psychopathologisation as a personal, portable psychiatric prison. *Discourse: Studies in the Cultural Politics of Education, 31*, 437–451.

Haslam, N. (2011). Genetic essentialism, neuroessentialism, and stigma: Commentary on Dar-Nimrod and Heine (2011). *Psychological Bulletin, 137*, 819–824.

Healy, D. (2008). Historical overview: Kraepelin's impact on psychiatry. *European Archives of Psychiatry and Clinical Neuroscience, 248*(Suppl 2), 18–24.

Hendriksen, J. (2009). *Handboek Intervisie [Intervision manual]*. Barneveld: Nelissen.

Highet, N., Stevenson, A. L., Purtell, C., & Coo, S. (2014). Qualitative insights into women's personal experiences of perinatal depression and anxiety. *Women and Birth, 27*, 179–184.

Hiller, W., Dichtl, G., Hecht, H., et al. (1993). An empirical comparison of diagnoses and reliabilities in ICD-10 and DSM-III-R. *European Archives of Psychiatry and Clinical Neuroscience, 242*, 209–217.

Husserl, E. (1950). *Cartesian meditations*. Dordrecht: Kluwer Academic Publishers.

Hyman, S. E. (2010). The diagnosis of mental disorders: The problem of reification. *Annual Review of Clinical Psychology, 6*, 155–179.

Insel, T. (2013). Transforming diagnosis. *Blogpost*. Retrieved December 10, 2013, from http://www.nimh.nih.gov/about/director/2013/transforming-diagnosis.shtml.

Insel, T., & Cuthbert, B. (2015). Brain disorders? Precisely. *Science, 348*, 499–500.

Insel, T. & Lieberman, J.A. (2013). DSM-5 and RDoC: Shared interests. *Blogpost*. Retrieved December 11, 2013, from http://www.nimh.nih.gov/news/science-news/2013/dsm-5-and-rdoc-shared-interests.shtml.

Insel, T., Cuthbert, B., Garvey, M., Heinssen, R., Pine, D.S.n., Quinn, K., Sanislow, C., & Wang, P. (2010). Research Domain Criteria (RDoC): Toward a new classification framework for research on mental disorders. *American Journal of Psychiatry, 167*, 748–751.

Jaspers, K. (1912). The phenomenological approach in psychopathology. *British Journal of Psychiatry, 114*, 1313–1323.

Jeste, D. V., Palmer, B. W., Rettew, D. C., & Boardman, S. (2015). Positive psychiatry: Its time has come. *Journal of Clinical Psychiatry, 76*, 675–683.

Kagan, J. (2012). *Psychology's ghosts – The crisis in the profession and the way back.* New Haven/London: Yale University Press.

Kahneman, D. (2011). *Thinking, fast and slow.* New York: Farra, Strauss & Giroux.

Kanfer, F. H., & Saslow, G. (1965). Behavioral analysis – An alternative to diagnostic classification. *Archives of General Psychiaty, 12*, 529–538.

Kant, E. (1764/2011). Essay on the maladies of the head. In P. Frierson & P. Cuyer (Eds.), *Emmanuel Kant: Observations on the feeling of the beautiful and sublime and other writings.* Cambridge: Cambridge University Press.

Kapur, S., Phillips, A. G., & Insel, T. R. (2012). Why has it taken so long for biological psychiatry to develop clinical tests and what to do about it? *Molecular Psychiatry, 17*, 1174–1179.

Karlsson, H. (2011). How psychotherapy changes the brain. *Psychiatric Times, 28*. Retrieved November 12, 2013, from http://www.psychiatrictimes.com/psychotherapy/how-psychotherapy-changes-brain.

Keim Campbell, J., O'Rourke, M., & Slater, M. H. (2011). *Carving nature at its joints: Natural kinds in metaphysics and science.* Cambridge: MIT Press.

Kelleher, I., Jenner, J., & Cannon, M. (2010). Psychotic symptoms in the general population – An evolutionary perspective. *British Journal of Psychiatry, 197*, 167–169.

Keller, M. B., Hanks, D. L., & Klein, D. N. (1996). Summary of the DSM-IV mood disorders field trial and issue overview. *The Psychiatric Clinics of North America, 19*, 1–28.

Kendler, K. S., Zachar, P., & Craver, C. (2011). What kinds of things are psychiatric disorders? *Psychological Medicine, 41*, 1143–1150.

Kirk, S. A., & Hsieh, D. K. (2004). Diagnostic consistency in assessing conduct disorder: An experiment on the effect of social context. *American Journal of Orthopsychiatry, 74*, 43–55.

Kirk, S. A., & Hsieh, D. K. (2009). Do perceptions of dysfunction and normality mediate clinicians judgments of adolescent antisocial behavior? *Social Service Review, 83*, 245–266.

Kirmayer, L. J., & Crafa, D. (2014). What kind of science for psychiatry. *Frontiers in Human Neuroscience, 8*, 435.

Kirshner, L. (2009). Biopolitics and the transformation of the psychiatric subject. In S. Binkley & J. Capetillo (Eds.), *A Foucault for the 21st century:*

Governmentality, biopolitics and discipline in the new millennium (pp. 92–104). Newcastle upon Tyne: Cambridge Scholars Publishing.

Klerman, G. L. (1978). The evolution of a scientific nosology. In J. C. Shershow (Ed.), *Schizophrenia: Science and practice* (pp. 99–121). New York/London: Guilford.

Kozak, M. J., & Cuthbert, B. N. (2016). The NIMH research domain criteria initiative: Background, issues and pragmatics. *Psychophysiology, 53*, 286–297.

Kraemer, H. C. (2015). Research Domain Criteria (RDoC) and the DSM – Two methodological approaches to mental health diagnosis. *JAMA Psychiatry, 72*, 1163–1164.

Kraemer, H. C., Periyakoil, V. S., & Noda, A. (2002). Tutorial in biostatistics: Kappa coefficients in medical research. *Statistical Medicine, 21*, 2109–2129.

Kraepelin, E. (1907). *Clinical psychiatry* (p. 1981). Delmar: Scholars' facsimiles and reprints.

Kraepelin, E. (1921). *Manic-depressive insanity and paranoia*. Edinburgh: Livingstone.

Kupfer, D. J., & Regier, D. A. (2011). Neuroscience, clinical evidence, and the future of psychiatric classification in DSM-5. *American Journal of Psychiatry, 168*, 672–674.

Kupfer, D. J., First, M. B., & Regier, D. A. (2002). *A research agenda for DSM-V*. Washington, DC: American Psychiatric Association.

Kutchins, H., & Kirk, S. A. (1997). *Making us crazy: DSM – The psychiatric bible and the creation of mental disorders*. New York: Free Press.

Kvaale, E. P., & Haslam, N. (2016). Motivational orientations and psychiatric stigma: Social motives influence how causal explanations relate to stigmatizing attitudes. *Personality and Individual Differences, 89*, 111–116.

Kvaale, E. P., Haslam, N., & Gottdiener, W. H. (2013). The 'side effects' of medicalization: A meta-analytic review of how biogenetic explanations affect stigma. *Clinical Psychology Review, 33*, 782–794.

Kvale, S. (1995). The social construction of validity. *Qualitative Inquiry, 1*, 19–40.

Lacan, J. (1964). *The seminar 1964, book XI, the four fundamental concepts of psycho-analysis*. London/New York: Karnac.

Lacan, J. (1975). Conférences et entretiens dans des universités nord-americaines [Conferences and interviews at North-American universities]. *Scilicet, 6/7*, 42–45.

Lacan, J. (1988 [1953–54]). *The seminar of Jacques Lacan, book I: Freud's papers on technique*. New York/London: W.W. Norton.

Lacan, J. (1988 [1954–55]). *The seminar of Jacques Lacan, book II, the ego in Freud's theory and in the technique of psychoanalysis*. Cambridge: Cambridge University Press.

Lacan, J. (1992 [1959–1960]). *The seminar, Book VII, the ethics of psychoanalysis*. London/New York: W. W. Norton.

Lacan, J. (2005 [1975–1976]). *Le séminaire, livre XXIII, le sinthome [The seminar, book XXIII, the sinthome]*. Paris: Seuil.

Lacan, J. (2006 [1947]). Presentation on psychical causality. In J. Lacan & J. A. Miller (Eds.), *Écrits* (pp. 123–158). New York/London: W. W. Norton.

Lacan, J. (2006 [1949]). The mirror stage as formative of the function of the I. In J. Lacan & J. A. Miller (Eds.), *Écrits* (pp. 75–81). New York/London: W. W. Norton.

Lacan, J. (2006 [1956a]). The situation of psychoanalysis and the training of psychoanalysts in 1956. In J. Lacan & J. A. Miller (Eds.), *Écrits* (pp. 384–411). New York/London: W. W. Norton.

Lacan, J. (1956b). Discours de Rome [The Rome discourse]. In J. Lacan (Ed.), *Autres Écrits* (pp. 133–165). Paris: Seuil.

Lacan, J. (2006 [1957]). The instance of the letter in the unconscious or reason since Freud. In J. Lacan & J. A. Miller (Eds.), *Écrits* (pp. 412–442). New York/London: W. W. Norton.

Lacan, J. (2006 [1959]). On a question prior to any possible treatment of psychosis. In J. Lacan & J. A. Miller (Eds.), *Écrits* (pp. 445–488). New York/London: W. W. Norton.

Lacan, J. (2006 [1961]). The direction of treatment and the principles of its power. In J. Lacan & J. A. Miller (Eds.), *Écrits* (pp. 489–542). New York/London: W. W. Norton.

Laing, R. D. (1960). *The divided self: An existential study in sanity and madness*. Harmondsworth: Penguin.

Landis, J. R., & Koch, G. G. (1977). The measurement of observer agreement for categorical data. *Biometrics, 33*, 159–174.

Lane, C. (2008). *Shyness: How normal behavior became sickness*. Yale: Yale University Press.

Laroi, F. (2012). How do auditory verbal hallucinations in patients differ from those in non-patients? *Frontiers in human neuroscience, 6*, 25.

Lévinas, E. (1982). La souffrance inutile [Pointless suffering]. In E. Lévinas (Ed.), *Entre nous. Essais sur le penser-à-l'autre* (pp. 100–112). Paris: Grasset, 1993.

Lévi-Strauss, C. (1958). *Antropologie structurale [Structural antrophology]*. Paris: Plon.

Lemaire, T. (2008). *Claude Lévi-Strauss. Tussen mythe en muziek [Claude Lévi-Strauss. In between myth and music]*. Amsterdam: Ambo.

Lilienfeld, S. O., & Marino, L. (1999). Essentialism revisited: Evolutionary theory and the concept of mental disorder. *Journal of Abnormal Psychology, 108*, 400–411.

Lincoln, Y. S., & Guba, E. G. (1985). *Naturalistic inquiry*. Newbury Park, CA: Sage.

Lindquist, K. A., Siegel, E. H., Quigley, K. S., & Battett, L. F. (2013). The hundred-year emotion way: Are emotions natural kinds or psychological constructions? Comment on Lench, Flores, and Bench (2011). *Psychological Bulletin, 139*, 255–263.

Madill, A., & Gough, B. (2008). Qualitative research and its place in psychological science. *Psychological Methods, 13*, 254–271.

Maj, M. (2012). Validity and clinical utility of the current operational characterization of major depression. *International Review of Psychiatry, 24*, 530–537.

Mallet, R., & Runswick-Cole, K. (2014). *Approaching disability: Critical issues and perspectives*. London/New York: Routledge.

Malterud, K. (2001). Qualitative research: Standards, challenges, and guidelines. *The Lancet, 358*, 483–488.

Marecek, J. (2003). Dancing through minefields: Towards a qualitative stance in psychology. In P. M. Camic, J. E. Rhodes, & L. Yardley (Eds.), *Qualtitative research in psychology* (pp. 49–69). Washington, DC: American Psychological Association.

Marková, I. S., & Berrios, G. E. (2009). Epistemology of mental symptoms. *Psychopathology, 42*, 343–349.

McNally, R. J. (2011). *What is mental illness?* Cambridge/London: Belknap Harvard.

Meehl, P. E. (1973). Why I do not attend case conferences. In *Psychodiagnosis: Selected papers* (pp. 225–302). Minneapolis: University of Minnesota Press.

Menninger, K. A. (1959). The psychiatric diagnosis. *Bulletin of the Menninger Clinic, 23*, 226–243.

Menninger, K., Ellenberger, H., Pruyser, P., & Mayman, M. (1958). The unitary concept of mental illness. *Bulletin of the Menninger Clinic, 22*, 4–12.

Merleau-Ponty, M. (1945). *La Phénoménologie de la Perception [The phenomenology of perception]*. Paris: Gallimard.

Miles, M., & Huberman, M. (1994). *Qualitative data analysis*. London: Sage.

Miller, J. A. (1983). Pas de Clinique sans éthique [No clinic without ethics]. *Actes de l'ECF, 5*, 65–68.

Miller, S., Hubble, M., & Duncan, B. (2007). Supershrinks – What's the secret of their success? *Psychotherapy Networker, 31*(6).

Moore, J. (2001). On distinguishing methodological from radical behaviorism. *European Journal of Behavioral Analysis, 2*, 221–244.

Mor Barak, M. E., Travis, D. J., Pyun, H., & Xie, B. (2009). The impact of supervision on worker outcomes: A meta-analysis. *The Social Service Review, 83*(1), 3–32.

Morse, J. M., Barrett, M., Mayan, M., Olson, K., & Spiers, J. (2002). Verification strategies for establishing reliability and validity in qualitative research. *International Journal of Qualitative Methods, 1*(2), Article 2.

Moskowitz, A., & Heim, G. (2011). Eugen Bleuler's Dementia praecox or the group of Schizophrenias (1911): A centenary appreciation and reconsideration. *Schizophrenia Bulletin, 37*, 471–479.

Moynihan, R., Heath, I., & Henry, D. (2002). Selling sickness: The pharmaceutical industry and disease mongering. Commentary: Medicalisation of risk factors. *BMJ, 324*, 886–891.

Mukolo, A., Heflinger, C. A., & Wallston, K. A. (2010). The stigma of childhood mental disorders: A conceptual framework. *Journal of the American Academy of Child and Adolescent Psychiatry, 49*, 92–198.

Nietsche, F. (1887). *The gay science*. New York: Vintage Books.

Nieweg, E. H. (2005). On reification and natural kinds in psychiatry. *Tijdschrift voor Psychiatrie, 47*, 687–696.

Nobus, D. (2000). *Jacques Lacan and the Freudian practice of psychoanalysis*. New York: Routledge.

O'Loughlin, M., Charles, M., Crosby, J., et al. (2014). Closing the gap: Narrating the prose of severe psychic suffering. *Psychoanalysis, Culture & Society, 19*, 98–106.

Orbach, I., Mikulincer, M., Sirota, P., et al. (2003). Mental pain: A multidimensional operationalization and definition. *Suicide and Life-Threatening Behavior, 33*, 219–230.

Parens, E., & Johnston, J. (2011). Troubled children: Diagnosing, treating and attending to context: A hastings center special report. *Hastings Center Report, 41*(2), S1–32.

Paris, J., & Kirmayer, L. J. (2016). The national institute of mental health research domain criteria: A bridge too far. *Journal of Nervous and Mental Disease, 204*, 26–32.

Parker, I. (2005). *Qualitative psychology: Introducing radical research*. Maidenhead/New York: Open University Press.

Parker, I. (2010). *Lacanian psychoanalysis – Revolutions on subjectivity*. London/New York: Routledge.

Parnas, J. (2012). The nature of the psychiatric object and classification. In K. S. Kendler & J. Parnas (Eds.), *Philosophical issues in psychiatry II – nosology* (pp. 118–123). Oxford: Oxford University Press.

Parnas, J., & Zahavi, D. (2000). The link: Philosophy-psychopathology-phenomenology. In D. Zahavi (Ed.), *Exploring the self*. Amsterdam: John Benjamins.

Pechey, R., & Halligan, P. (2011). The prevalence of delusion-like beliefs relative to sociocultural beliefs in the general population. *Psychopathology, 44*, 106–115.

Pechey, R., & Halligan, P. (2012). Prevalence and correlates of anomalous experiences in a large non-clinical sample. *Psychology and Psychotherapy: Theory, Research and Practice, 85*, 150–162.

Peerenboom, E. (2002). Transparent science. *EMBO Reports, 3*(1), 9–11.

Philips, C. B. (2006). Medicine goes to school: Teachers as sickness brokers for ADHD. *Plos Medicine, 3*, e182.

Pickard, H. (2009). Mental illness is indeed a myth. In L. Bortolotti & M. Broome (Eds.), *Psychiatry as cognitive science: Philosophical perspectives* (pp. 83–101). London: Open University Press.

Pigeaud, J. (2001). *Aux portes de la psychiatrie. Pinel, l'ancien et le moderne*. Paris: Aubier.

Pinel, P. (1806). *A treatise on insanity*. Sheffield: Todd.

Polkinghorne, D. (1990). Language and qualitative research. *Theoretical and Philosophical Psychology, 10*, 3–24.

Ponterotto, J. G. (2005). Qualitative research in counselling psychology: A primer on research paradigms and philosophy of science. *Journal of Counseling Psychology, 52*, 126–136.

Pottick, K. J., Kirk, S. A., Hsieh, D. K., & Tian, X. (2007). Judging mental disorder in youths: Effects of client, clinician and contextual factors. *Journal of Consulting and Clinical Psychology, 75*, 1–8.

Rafalovich, A. (2004). *Framing ADHD children: A critical examination of the history, discourse, and everyday experience of attention deficit/hyperactivity disorder*. Lanham: Lexington Books.

Réjon Altable, C. (2012). Logic structure of clinical judgment and its relation to medical and psychiatric semiology. *Psychopathology, 45*, 344–351.

Regier, D. A., Narrow, W. E., Kuhl, E. A., & Kupfer, D. J. (2009). The conceptual development of DSM-V. *American Journal of Psychiatry, 166*, 645–650.

Regier, D. A., Narrow, W. E., Clarke, D. E., et al. (2013). DSM-5 field trials in the United States and Canada, part II: Test-retest reliability of selected categorical diagnoses. *American Journal of Psychiatry, 170*, 59–70.

Reynolds, C. F., Lewis, D. A., Detre, T., Schatzberg, A. F., & Kupfer, D. J. (2009). The future of psychiatry as clinical neuroscience. *Academic Medicine, 84*, 446–450.

Richardson, L. (1994). Writing: A method of inquiry. In N. K. Denzin & Y. S. Lincoln (Eds.), *Handbook of qualitative research* (pp. 516–529). Thousand Oaks: Sage.

Robins, E., & Guze, S. (1970). Establishment of diagnostic validity in psychiatric illness: Its application to schizophrenia. *American Journal of Psychiatry, 126*, 983–987.

Rose, N. (1996). *Inventing our selves – Psychology, power and personhood*. Cambridge: Cambridge University Press.

Rose, N. (1999). *Governing the soul – The shaping of the private self – Second edition*. London/New York: Free Association Books.

Rosen, G. M., & Lilienfeld, S. O. (2008). Posttraumatic stress disorder: An empirical evaluation of core assumptions. *Clinical Psychology Review, 28*, 837–868.

Rosenhan, D. (1973). Being sane in insane places. *Science, 179*, 250–258.

Rosenhan, D. (1975). The contextual nature of psychiatric diagnosis. *Journal of Abnormal Psychology, 84*, 462–474.

Sandifer, M. S., Hordern, A., & Green, L. M. (1970). The psychiatric interview: The impact of the first three minutes. *American Journal of Psychiatry, 126*, 968–973.

Schacter, D. L. (1999). The seven sins of memory: Insights from psychology and cognitive neuroscience. *American Psychologist, 54*, 182–203.

Scheff, T. (1966). *Being mentally ill – A sociological theory*. Chicago: Aldine.

Schomerus, G., Schwahn, C., Holzinger, A., et al. (2012). Evolution of public attitudes about mental illness: A systematic review and meta-analysis. *Acta Psychiatrica Scandinavica, 125*, 440–452.

Seikkula, J., Aaltonen, J., Alakare, B., et al. (2006). Five-year experience of first-episode nonaffective psychosis open-dialogue approach: Treatment principles, follow-up outcomes and two case studies. *Psychotherapy Research, 16*, 214–228.

Showalter, E. (1998). *Hystories*. New York: Columbia University Press.

Skre, I., Onstad, S., Torgensen, S., & Kringlen, E. (1991). High interrater reliability for the structured clinical interview for DSM-III-R Axis I (SCID-I). *Acta Psychiatrica Scandinavica, 84*, 167–173.

Solomon, A. (2012). *Far from the tree – Parents, children and the search for identity*. London: Vintage books.

Spitzer, R. L. (1975). On pseudoscience in science, logic in remission and psychiatric diagnosis: A critique of Rosenhan's 'on being sane in insane places'. *Journal of Abnormal Psychology, 84*, 442–452.

Spitzer, R. L., & Fleiss, J. L. (1974). A re-analysis of the reliability of psychiatric diagnosis. *British Journal of Psychiatry, 125*, 341–347.

Spitzer, R. L., Endicot, J., & Robins, E. (1978). Research diagnostic criteria – Rationale and reliability. *Archives of General Psychiatry, 35*, 773–782.

Spitzer, R. L., Forman, J. B. W., & Nee, J. (1979). DSM-III field trials: I. Initial interrater diagnostic reliability. *American Journal of Psychiatry, 136*, 815–817.

Spitzer, R. L., Williams, J. B., Gibbon, M., & First, M. B. (1984). *Structured clinical interview for DSM-III axis I disorders*. New York: New York State Psychiatric Institute.

Stein, D. J., Phillips, K. A., Bolton, D., Fulford, K. W. M., Sadler, J. S., & Kendler, K. S. (2010). What is a mental/psychiatric disorder? From DSM-IV to DSM-V. *Psychological Medicine, 40*, 1759–1765.

Stiles, W. B. (1993). Quality control in qualitative research. *Clinical Psychology Review, 13*, 593–618.

Stoyanov, D., Machamer, P. K., Schaffner, K. F., & Rivera-Hernández, R. (2012). The challenge of psychiatric nosology and diagnosis. *Journal of Evaluation in Clinical Practice, 18*, 704–709.

Strand, M. (2011). Where do classifications come from? The DSM-III, the transformation of American psychiatry, and the problem of origins in the sociology of knowledge. *Theory and Society, 40*, 273–313.

Sturmey, P. (2009). Case formulation: A review and overview of this volume. In P. Sturmey (Ed.), *Clinical case formulation: Varieties of approaches* (pp. 3–32). Oxford: Wiley-Blackwell.

Szasz, T. S. (1961). *The myth of mental illness – Foundations of the theory of personal conduct.* New York: Harper & Row.

Tait, G. (2009). The logic of ADHD: A brief review of fallacious reasoning. *Studies in Philosophy and Education, 28*, 239–254.

Temerlin, M. K. (1968). Suggestion effects in psychiatric diagnosis. *Journal of Nervous and Mental Disease, 147*, 349–353.

Temerlin, M. K. (1970). Diagnostic bias in community mental health. *Community Mental Health Journal, 6*, 110–117.

The Psychologist. (2011). Society's critical response to DSM-5. Retrieved Oktober 17, 2013, from http://www.thepsychologist.org.uk/blog/blogpost.cfm?threadid=2102&catid=48.

Timimi, S., & Leo, J. (2009). *Rethinking ADHD*. London/New York: Palgrave MacMillan.

Trajkovic, G., Starcevic, V., Latas, M., et al. (2011). Reliability of the Hamilton rating scale for depression: A meta-analysis over a period of 49 years. *Psychiatry Research, 189*, 1–9.

Trudgen, R. (2000). *Why warriors lie down and die. Towards an understanding of why the Aboriginal people of Arnhem land face the greatest crisis in health and education since European contact.* Darwin: Aboriginal Resource and Developmental Services Inc.

Van Os, J. (2010). Are psychiatric diagnoses of psychosis scientific and useful? The case of schizophrenia. *Journal of Mental Health, 19*, 305–317.

Van Os, J. (2016). "Schizophrenia" does not exist. *The British Medical Journal, 352*, i375.

Van Os, J., Kenis, G., & Rutten, B. P. (2010). The environment and schizophrenia. *Nature, 268*, 203–212.

Van Os, J., Rutten, B. P., Myin-Germeys, I., et al. (2014). Identifying gene-environment interactions in schizophrenia: Contemporary challenges for integrated, large-scale investigations. *Schizophrenia Bulletin, 40*, 729–736.

Van Roy, K., Vanheule, S., Debaere, V., Inslegers, R., Meganck, R., & Deganck, J. (2014). A Lacanian view on Balint group meetings: A qualitative analysis of two case presentations. *BMC Family Practice, 15*, 49. doi:10.1186/1471-2296-15-49.

Vanheule, S. (2011). *The subject of psychosis – A Lacanian perspective.* London/New York: Palgrave MacMillan.

Vanheule, S. (2012). Diagnosis in the field of psychotherapy: A plea for an alternative to the DSM-5.x. *Psychology and Psychotherapy: Theory, Research and Practice, 85*, 128–142.

Vanheule, S., & Devisch, I. (2014). Mental suffering and the DSM-5: A critical review. *The Journal of Evaluation of Clinical Practice, 20*, 975–980.

Vanheule, S., & Verhaeghe, P. (2004). Powerlessness and impossibility in special education: A qualitative study on professional burnout from a Lacanian perspective. *Human Relations, 57*, 497–519.

Vanheule, S., Lievrouw, A., & Verhaeghe, P. (2003). Burnout and intersubjectivity: A psychoanalytical study from a Lacanian perspective. *Human Relations, 56*, 321–339.

Vanheule, S., Desmet, M., Meganck, R., et al. (2014). Reliability in psychiatric diagnosis with the DSM: Old wine in new barrels. *Psychotherapy and Psychosomatics, 83*, 313–314.

Verhaeghe, P. (2002). *On being normal and other disorders.* New York: Other Press.

Verhaeghe, P. (2014). *What about me? – The struggle for identity in a market-based society*. Victoria/London: Scribe.

Vertue, F. M., & Haig, B. D. (2008). An abductive perspective on clinical reasoning and case formulation. *Journal of Clinical Psychology, 64*, 1046–1068.

Viera, A. J., & Garrett, J. M. (2005). Understanding interobserver agreement: The kappa statistic. *Family Medicine, 37*, 360–363.

Wakefield, J. C. (1992). Disorder as harmful dysfunction: A conceptual critique of DSM-II-R's definition of mental disorder. *Psychological Review, 99*, 232–247.

Wakefield, J. C. (2010). Misdiagnosing normality: Psychiatry's failure to address the problem of false positive diagnoses of mental disorder in a changing professional environment. *Journal of Mental Health, 19*, 337–351.

Watt, D. (2007). On becoming a qualitative researcher: The value of reflexivity. *The Qualitative Report, 12*, 82–101.

Watters, E. (2010). *Crazy like us: The globalization of the American psyche*. New York: Free Press.

Weber, M. M., & Engstrom, E. J. (1997). Kraepelin's "diagnostic cards". The confluence of clinical research and preconceived categories. *History of Psychiatry, 8*, 375–385.

Weinberger, D. R., Glick, I. D., & Klein, D. F. (2015). Whither Research Domain Criteria (RDoC)? The good, the bad, and the ugly. *JAMA Psychiatry, 72*, 1161–1162.

Welner, A., Liss, J. L., & Robins, E. (1974). Systematic approach for making a psychiatric diagnosis. *Archives of General Psychiatry, 31*, 193–196.

Westen, D. (2012). Protoype diagnosis of psychiatric syndromes. *World Psychiatry, 11*, 16–21.

Westen, D., DeFife, J. A., Bradley, B., & Hilsenroth, M. J. (2010). Prototype personality diagnosis in clinical practice: A viable alternative for DSM-5 and ICD-11. *Professional Psychology: Research and Practice, 41*, 482–487.

Whiteford, H. A., Degenhardt, L., Rehm, J., et al. (2013). Global burden of disease attributable to mental and substance use disorders: Findings from the Global Burden of Disease Study 2010. *The Lancet, 382*, 1575–1586.

Wigman, J. T. W., van Os, J., Thiery, E., et al. (2013). Psychiatric diagnosis revisited: Towards a system of staging and profiling combining nomothetic and idiographic parameters of momentary mental states. *PLoS ONE, 8*, e59559.

Wilkinson, R. G., & Pickett, L. (2009). *The spirit level: Why more equal societies almost always do better*. London: Allan Lane.

Williams, J. B. W., & Kobak, K. A. (2008). Development and reliability of a structured interview guide for the montgomery depression rating scale (SIGMA). *British Journal of Psychiatry, 192*, 52–58.

Williams, J. B. W., Gibbon, M., First, M. B., et al. (1992). The structured clinical interview for DSM-III-R (SCID) – II. Multisite test-retest reliability. *Archives of General Psychiatry, 49*, 630–636.

Woodruff, R., Goodwin, D., & Guze, S. (1974). *Psychiatric diagnosis*. New York: Oxford University Press.

World Health Organization. (2010). *Measuring health and disability: Manual for WHO Disability Assessment Schedule (WHODAS 2.0)*. Geneva: World Health Organization.

World Health Organization. (2011a). *World report on disability*. Geneva: World Health Organization.

World Health Organization. (2011b). *World report on disability – Summary*. Geneva: World Health Organization.

World Health Organization. (2012). Global burden of mental disorders and the need of a comprehensive, coordinated response from health and social sectors at the country level. Sixty-Fifth Wold Health Assembly. Geneva: World Health Organization. Retrieved October 4, 2013, from http://apps.who.int/gb/ebwha/pdf_files/WHA65/A65_10-en.pdf.

World Health Organization. (2013). Mental health action plan 2013–2020. Geneva: World Health Organization. Retrieved June 21, 2016, from http://apps.who.int/iris/bitstream/10665/89966/1/9789241506021_eng.pdf.

Wundt, W. (1897). *Outlines of psychology*. Leipzig: Wilhelm Engelman.

Zachar, P. (2002). The practical kinds model as a pragmatist theory of classification. *Philosophy, Psychology and Psychiatry, 9*, 219–227.

Zanarini, M. C., Skodol, A. E., Bender, D., et al. (2000). The collaborative longitudinal personality disorders study: Reliability of Axis I and II diagnoses. *Journal of Personality Disorders, 14*, 291–299.

Ziółkowska, J. (2012). The objectifying discourse of doctors' questions. Qualitative analysis of psychiatric interviews. *Social Theory & Health, 10*, 292–307.

Index

A

abductive reasoning, 162, 163, 173
abnormality, 4, 5, 19, 136, 138–44, 153, 154, 157, 163
ad hoc fallacy, 18, 20
affective disorders, 25, 27, 48, 49, 53, 61
alcoholism, 24, 25, 49, 67
alcohol use disorder, 11, 11n1, 60, 68, 85
alienation, 35, 190n4
American Medico-Psychological Association, 12
American Psychiatric Association (APA), 1, 2, 12, 13, 15, 86, 106
Andreasen, Nancy, 82
anti-psychiatry, 189
Aspies For Freedom, 37
asylums, 31
attention deficit hyperactivity disorder (ADHD), 32, 35, 38, 41, 61, 63, 109n10, 133, 134, 139, 155
autism, 37, 38, 61, 85

B

Bacon, Francis, 182
Balint groups, 193
Balint, Michael, 193
Barnum effect, 18
Bayle, Antoine Laurent, 121
Beavan, V., 91
Beck, Aaron, 26
bell curve, 141
Bergmann, J., 34, 35
Bernstein, Carol A., 106, 109, 122

Note: Page number followed by 'n' refers to notes

Berrios, German, 4, 45, 46, 85, 93–6, 98, 100, 106, 108, 109, 115, 126, 160, 168, 184
beware of understanding, 5, 161, 184
bias, 33, 68, 184, 197–9
biomarkers, 116
biomedical model, 27, 30
biomedical referents, 105–10
biopolitics, 138
biopsychological focus, 111, 113, 115, 119
biopsychopathology, 110–18, 126
biosignatures bipolar disorder, 55, 63, 64, 112, 116
blame, 36
Bleuler, Eugen, 10, 11
Borsboom, D., 93n5, 171
brain, 14, 24–6, 33, 46, 47, 60, 94–7, 106, 108, 109, 111, 112, 115, 116, 120, 121, 123, 145
Breuer, Joseph, 172
Bruner, Jerome, 148, 176–8
burnout, 187

C

Cambridge model of symptom formation, 94–9, 103, 105, 116, 118
Canguilhem, Georges, 113, 138–40, 142–4, 161, 162
cartels, 191–3, 196, 199, 204
case constructions, 3, 5, 6, 152, 153, 161–3, 171–3, 184, 195, 196, 199, 202, 203, 205
case formulation, 2, 5, 6, 81–4, 89, 152, 153, 158, 162, 163, 167–207

Cassell, Eric, 148, 150, 151
casuistic approach, 4, 80, 125
casuistic description, 171
categorical classification, 12, 13
census studies, 12
characteristics, 4, 5, 9–11, 16, 19, 32, 33, 69, 80, 85, 87, 89, 90, 92, 95, 99–102, 103n6, 104, 105, 109, 111, 117, 122, 124, 125, 137, 139, 141, 143–5, 150, 152–4, 161, 162, 172, 180, 185, 187, 188, 197, 202
Charney, Dennis, 115
checklist-based diagnosis, 3, 26
Chmielewski, M., 63–7
Clarke, D.E., 22–5, 27, 48, 49, 53, 54, 56–61, 63–6
classificatory systems, 2, 13
clinical case formulation, 2, 5, 6, 81, 82, 89, 153, 167–207
clinical decision-making
criticism of, 18, 113
transparency in, 197, 199
clinical diary, 190, 191
clinical judgment, 81
clinical meetings, 171, 174, 195, 199, 205
clinical notes, 195–7, 199, 203
clinical reasoning, 70
clinical structures, 103, 104, 126, 206
clinical vignettes, 10
comorbidity rates, 62
complexity, 171, 178, 190, 203
Compton, W.M., 45, 46
configuration processes, 94, 96, 97, 102, 103, 105, 116, 118, 162, 168

conflict, 15, 42, 88, 150, 154, 156, 162, 175
consumption, 2, 39, 41
context
  in DSM, 84
  individual, 4, 79, 81
conversation analytic studies, 34
Cooper, Rachel, 113, 119, 120, 123, 124, 137, 138, 143, 155
Cosgrove, L., 42
credibility, 2, 5, 20, 26, 43, 50, 67, 69, 110, 126, 200–2
criterion-based diagnosis, 8, 48
critical researchers, 4, 28–40, 122
cultural case formulation, 81–3
Cultural Formulation Interview (CFI), 81, 83

D

Decker, Hannah, 15, 26, 27, 40, 44–6, 50, 51, 82, 90n3, 105, 106, 158
deinstitutionalization, 40–4
de la Mettrie, Julien Offray, 176
delusional beliefs, 91
dementia praecox, 46, 109
demonstrative cases, 10
de Saussure, Ferdinand, 98, 102
descriptive criteria, 7, 106
deviance, 141, 154–6
diagignoskein, 13
diagnosis
  biomedical referents, 105–10
  brain marker, 33
  casuistic approach to, 4, 80, 125
  checklist-based, 3, 8, 26
  as classification, 2, 3, 90, 167, 187
  context and, 155

credibility of, 20, 126
criterion-based, 8, 40, 48
criticism of psychiatric, 47, 159, 170
decision-making, 8–70
descriptive-based, 84–7
false-positive, 20, 44, 50
fashions, 188
function-oriented, 169–72, 174, 199, 202, 204–7
idea of, 79
influence of pharmaceutical industry on, 42
polythetic descriptive, 84–7
power, 107
prototype-based, 8, 28, 86
reification and, 39
reliability of, 107
Rosenhan study of, 21
signed-based, 87–101
stigma and, 4, 34, 36, 39
Temerlin study on, 18
Diagnostic and Statistical Manual of Mental Disorders (DSM), 1–8, 10–14, 14n2, 27, 28, 31–4, 40–2, 44, 51, 52, 55, 59, 62, 67–70, 79–90, 93, 94, 96, 104, 105, 108, 122, 123, 125, 133, 134, 154–8, 167–9, 171, 205–7
  development of, 13
Diagnostic and Statistical Manual of Mental Disorders, Fifth Edition (DSM-5), 2–5, 7, 8, 10, 11, 11n1, 15, 23, 23n4, 27, 42–4, 51, 52, 55, 59–62, 62n15, 63, 64, 80, 81, 83–6, 88, 89, 92, 106, 107, 107n9, 108, 109, 109n10, 110,

110n11, 112, 115, 121–3, 125, 133, 139, 140, 151, 153–8, 168, 206
  context and, 4
Diagnostic and Statistical Manual of Mental Disorders, Fifth Edition (DSM-5) diagnostic categories in, 62
Diagnostic and Statistical Manual of Mental Disorders, Fifth Edition (DSM-5) field trials, 8, 23, 27, 52, 59–64
Diagnostic and Statistical Manual of Mental Disorders, Fifth Edition (DSM-5) reliability of, 3
Diagnostic and Statistical Manual of Mental Disorders, Fifth Edition (DSM-5) severity assessment in, 10
Diagnostic and Statistical Manual of Mental Disorders, First Edition (DSM-I), 8, 11, 13–15, 54, 105
Diagnostic and Statistical Manual of Mental Disorders, Fourth Edition (DSM-IV), 42, 51, 58, 59, 64, 106, 107, 122
Diagnostic and Statistical Manual of Mental Disorders, Second Edition (DSM-II), 11, 11n2, 15, 21, 22, 25, 26, 30, 50, 54, 158
Diagnostic and Statistical Manual of Mental Disorders, Third Edition (DSM-III)
  descriptive approach in, 86, 106
  development of, 26
  field trials, 53, 54

reliability of, 8, 16, 26, 27, 52, 55, 67
diagnostic criteria, 10, 33, 47–9, 51, 55n11, 58, 59, 61, 81, 82, 107, 109, 134, 139, 140
diagnostic labeling, 38
dialogical interventions, 147
disability, 1, 11, 113, 145, 154, 156–8, 167, 169
disciplinary power, 31, 34
disciplining, 39, 142
discourse analysis, 179
disease mongering, 41
distortion, 179, 197–9
diversity, 85, 139, 140, 178, 179
doctor-patient relationship, 34
Dora, 169, 173
DSM. *See* Diagnostic and Statistical Manual of Mental Disorders
dysfunction, 51, 54, 111, 153–7

E

Eco, Umberto, 88
empathic accuracy, 160, 161
empowerment, 157
epistemic prison, 32
essentialist kinds, 120, 123
ethical values, 135
ethics of the lack, 135
exclusion, 41, 42, 69, 80, 84, 85, 88, 107, 109n10, 157
existential questions, 104
extimate element, 149

F

false-negative diagnosis, 20, 50
false-positive diagnosis, 20, 50

Feighner, John, 45, 47, 48, 50
Ferenczi, Sándor, 191
Fleiss, Joseph, 21–7, 30, 48, 49, 53, 54, 56–61, 63–6
Foucault, Michel, 28, 30, 31, 34, 35, 39, 68, 138, 182, 188, 189
Frances, A., 1, 42, 63, 109n10, 110, 140
Freedman, R., 62
Freud, Sigmund, 92, 145, 169, 170, 173, 185, 186, 186n3, 195, 196

G

gardez-vous de comprendre, 5, 158–61, 161n2, 184
gaze, 36, 183
general paralysis, 121
genetic essentialism, 33, 108
genetic studies, 32
genuine understanding, 5, 159
Georget, 108
Goclenius, Rudolph, 140
good listening, 135, 136
Grob, G.N., 12, 13, 40
Guze, Samuel, 45–7, 50

H

Hacking, Ian, 119, 120, 124
Hammerslag, Anna, 185, 186
Harwood, Valerie, 38
heterophenomenological approach, 117
Highet, Nicole, 174, 175
homosexuality, 37, 48, 139, 158
human kinds, 124

Husserl, Edmund, 118
Hyman, Steven, 31, 32, 34, 51, 63, 122
hysterical complaints, 29, 30

I

ideal-ego, 39
identification, 37, 45, 97, 160, 161
identity categories, 37
idiosyncrasies, 69, 157, 163, 197
Imaginary, 5, 102, 103, 117, 160, 161
indexical signifiers, 88
individual context, 4, 79, 81
individual speaking, 98
insanity, 9, 30, 46
insurance agencies, 41
International Classification of Diseases (ICD), 15
The Interpretation of Dreams, 138, 185, 186
inter-rater reliability, 21, 24, 27, 28, 30, 57, 62, 67
interview, 16, 17, 46, 48, 55, 64, 67, 81–3, 87, 142, 179, 182, 195
intrusion, 35
Irma, 185, 186n3

J

Jaspers, Karl, 159, 160
Johnston, Josephine, 63, 134, 135
The Jokes and their Relation to the Unconscious, 138
jouissance, 147, 149, 162
Joyce, James, 152

K

Kant, Immanuel, 9
kappa coefficients, 22, 23, 25–7, 49, 52–4, 56, 56n13, 57–61, 61n14, 62–7
Kirk, S.A., 8, 50, 51, 56, 158
knot theory, 152
knowledge, 13, 17, 19, 26, 35, 45, 69, 79, 83, 95, 100, 101, 118, 124, 162, 167, 173–5, 182, 183, 188, 203, 204
Koch, G.G., 23–7, 48, 49, 53, 54, 56–61, 65, 66
Kozak, M.J., 110–13, 115–18
Kraepelin, Emil, 10, 12, 45
Kupfer, David, 107, 108, 110, 110n11, 112
Kutchins, H., 8, 56, 158

L

Lacanian psychoanalysis, 4, 104n7
Lacan, Jacques, 44, 68, 97, 101, 102, 118, 135, 136, 150, 152, 160, 161, 176, 184, 189, 190n4, 192n5, 193
Laing, Ronald, 28
Landis, J.R., 23–7, 48, 49, 53, 54, 56–61, 65, 66
language, 2, 7, 29, 31, 34, 35, 87, 95, 98–102, 114, 133, 145, 152, 162, 175, 177–9, 206
language-use, 35, 98, 102, 179
Lanzer, Ernst, 195
laypersons, 17, 34, 88, 90
Leriche, René, 161
Lévinas, Emmanuel, 160
Lévi-Strauss, Claude, 183
Lilienfeld, Scott, 63, 86, 122

M

madman, 30, 31
madness, 30, 31, 102, 109, 152
major depressive disorder, 42, 49, 60, 61, 64–6, 84–7
maladaptation, 139
Markova, Ivana, 4, 93–6, 98, 100, 106, 108, 109, 115, 126, 168, 184
materialism, 104n7
mechanistic property clusters (MPC), 123
medical doctors, 31
medical model, 36, 46. *See also* biomedical model
medical semiotics, 88, 125
Meehl, Paul, 18–20, 39, 69, 184, 199, 204
Menninger, Karl, 12, 14, 15, 32
mental derangement, forms of, 9
mental disorders
　biomedical model of, 30
　categories of, 32, 111
　definition of, 83, 153, 157, 158
　description of, 11, 14, 86, 159
　as essentialist kinds, 120
　genetic studies on, 32
　increase in, 14, 14n3
　as natural kinds, 119n13
　as practical kinds, 122
　as reflexive kinds, 124
mental health, 1–3, 8, 11, 13, 17, 32, 36–8, 40, 41, 44, 65, 67, 83, 91, 114, 124, 126, 137, 145, 152, 156, 159, 162, 163, 167–9, 180, 189, 190, 196, 207
mental health care
　changes in, 40, 44
　rationalization of, 41

mental pain, 136, 145, 147
mental symptoms. *See* symptoms
methodological marginalization, 183
me-too fallacy, 18
Miles, M., 194, 197–201
mobile asylum, 38
moral evaluation, 143
morality, 35
Morse, J.M., 194, 195, 197

N

narrative approach, 3, 178
National Institute of Mental Health (NIMH), 32, 110, 112, 123, 126
naturalistic, 14, 16, 50, 93, 123, 126, 194
natural kinds, 31, 107, 119, 120, 122–4, 126
neo-Kraepelinians, 16, 45–7, 50, 68
neo-liberal society, 39
neopositivism, 88
neurodiversity, 37
neuroessentialism, 33, 108
neurosis, 17, 18, 25–7, 48, 103, 105, 195
Nietzsche, Friedrich, 31
Noguchi, Hideyo, 121
nomenclature, 12, 26
normal distribution, 12, 26

O

ontological transmutation, 16

P

paradigmatic thinking, 187, 188
paranormal experiences, 91
Parens, Eric, 63, 134, 135
Parker, Ian, 84n1, 103, 178, 181, 182
Parnas, Josef, 90, 93, 159
participant observation, 182
particularities, 47, 103, 103n6, 105, 124, 204
pathos, 5, 136, 142–51, 153, 157, 158, 162
Pechey, R., 91
peer debriefing, 201, 203
personality disorders, 14, 25, 26, 28, 54, 55, 57, 59, 60
perversion, 103, 139
pessimism, 36
pharmaceutical industry, 2, 40–2
phenomenological, 4, 5, 62n15, 90n3, 91n4, 118, 159, 160, 179
phenomenology, 144
philosophical, 91n4, 92n4, 122, 137
philosophy, 119
Pickard, Hanna, 30
Pinel, Philippe, 9
polythetic descriptive diagnosis, 84–7
population norms, 137
positivism, 31
post-traumatic stress disorder (PTSD), 60, 62–4
power-related regimes, 34
power relations, 31, 136, 179
practical kinds, 122, 123
pragmatic approach, 80
preconceptions, 174, 181, 183, 185, 197
prejudice, 17, 18, 36, 37, 70, 156, 157, 186
process-thinking, 29, 39
prognosis, 9, 10, 36, 45, 113

prototype-based diagnosis, 8, 28, 86n2
prototype-matching, 28
psychiatric expertise, 35
psychiatric institutions, 40
psychiatric statistics, 12
psychiatric symptoms, 19, 29, 114, 146n1
psychiatrizing focus, 134
psychiatry
  biomedical model of, 27
  changes in, 3, 8
  criticism of, 12, 21, 34, 36, 44, 160
  disease mongering in, 41
  ethos of, 3, 8, 36
  as medical discipline, 3, 15, 46
  standard nomenclature for, 12
psychical causality, 97, 98
psychic pain, 145, 146n1
psychoanalysis, 4, 15, 27, 30n6, 45, 104n7, 105, 190, 190n4, 191
psychoanalysts, 26, 44, 171, 182, 190n4, 191
psychoanalytic therapy, 13
psychodynamic theory, 15
psychological assessment, 39, 142
psychopathology
  biomedical model of, 27, 30
  classification of, 110
The Psychopathology of Everyday Life, 138
psychosis, 11n2, 17, 19, 21, 25–7, 33, 44, 46, 63, 64, 103, 147
psychotherapeutic, 41, 107, 172
psychotherapy, 97, 172, 190, 191
psychotic, 14, 16, 17, 24n5, 25, 42, 55, 65, 66, 80, 91, 104
psychotropic medications, 40

psy-professionals, 17, 35, 83, 92, 175, 187–90, 206

Q

qualitative inquiry, 176, 178, 179
qualitative research, 5, 174–82, 185, 187, 190, 194, 197–201, 203–5
quality assurance, 179–80
quality of mental suffering, 5, 150
Quetelet, Adolphe, 141

R

randomized controlled trials, 41
rationalization, 40–4
Real, 5, 101–3, 104n7, 105, 117, 125, 152, 187
recovery, 114, 161
referents, 88–90, 105–10, 112
reflexive kinds, 124, 125
reflexive relations, 90–2, 104n7, 116, 125
reflexivity
  institutional, 181, 183, 185, 187, 191, 193
  personal, 185
  relational, 179, 183, 185, 191, 193
Regier, Darrel, 44, 51, 59–63, 107, 108, 110n11, 112, 121
regime of truth, 35
reification, 4, 31–4, 37, 39, 68, 80, 116, 120
reliability
  in diagnosis, 21, 22, 26, 48, 50, 52–68, 112
  inter-rater, 21, 24, 27, 28, 30, 57, 62, 67

test-retest, 55, 59, 114
A Research Agenda for DSM-V, 107
research audit, 198, 199, 201
Research Diagnostic Criteria (RDC), 48–50
research diary, 181–3, 190
Research Domain Criteria (RDoC) report, 110–19, 123, 126
responsibility, 36
rhetorical, 34, 108, 169
Ricoeur, Paul, 144, 146, 148, 149
Robins, Eli, 45, 47, 50
Roschian concept, 86
Rosen, Gerald, 63
Rosenhan, David, 19, 20, 68
Rose, Nikolas, 38, 39, 84n1, 142
rule-breaking communications, 30

S

Saint Martin of Tours, 135
Scheff, Thomas, 28
schizo-affective disorder, 49, 55, 56, 60, 63, 85
schizophrenia, 10, 11, 14, 19, 25, 32, 33, 42, 48, 49, 55, 56, 60, 63, 80, 85–7, 111
self-advocacy, 37
self-experience, 91n4, 101, 103, 147–9
self-government, 39
self-reflexivity, 91n4, 92n4, 150
semiotic theory, 88, 90
severity assessment, 10
sick-sick fallacy, 18, 19
sign-based diagnosis, 87–101
signified, 90, 101, 102, 104, 170n1, 171

signifiers, 88–90, 91n4, 92n4, 101, 102, 104, 116, 126, 150, 170n1, 171
signs, 10, 21, 29, 43, 66, 79, 84, 88–90, 93, 95, 98, 99, 105, 109, 112, 114, 125, 135, 145, 154, 186n3
singularities, 103–5, 103n6, 124, 203, 204, 206
social adaptation, 140
social norms, 36, 39, 142
social physics, 141
social psychiatry, 107
soldiers, 13, 135
Solomon, Andrew, 37
soul, 39, 145
speech, 35, 86, 91n4, 92n4, 98–104, 116, 118, 147, 151, 159, 175
speech act, 4, 98–102, 116, 118
Spitzer, Robert, 21–7, 30, 43, 46, 48–50, 52–61, 63–6, 82, 158
Statistical Manual for the Use of Institutions for the Insane, 12–14, 70
statistics, 12, 13, 23, 26
Stein, D.J., 107
stereotyping, 38
stigma, 4, 34, 36, 37, 39
stories, 68, 148, 177, 178, 200
Strand, M., 11, 13, 14, 16, 40, 41, 45, 46
Structural Clinical Interview for DSM (SCID), 55, 55n12, 57, 59, 63–5, 87
subject, 3, 9, 29, 35, 70, 90, 91, 91n4, 92, 92n4, 101, 104n7, 116, 118, 124, 125, 168, 182, 189, 190n4, 193, 203

subjective logic, 171, 174
subjectivism, 117
subjectivity, 39, 68, 69, 91n4, 92n4, 93, 117, 118, 138, 142, 168, 177, 178, 183, 186
suffering, 1, 5, 7, 8, 11, 14, 17, 45, 66, 84, 90, 94, 101, 103, 104, 116, 117, 133–63, 167–9, 170n1, 189, 196
supervision, 5, 69, 191–3, 192n5, 196, 199, 203
Sydenham, Thomas, 9
symbolic, 5, 102, 103, 117, 124, 161
symptoms
    biomedical referents, 105–10
    Cambridge model, 94–9, 103, 105, 116, 118
    Lacan on, 101–5
    as personal constructions, 90–101
syndrome, 24, 25, 32, 44, 45, 53–5, 109, 111, 112, 121, 126, 150, 153, 154, 156, 162, 163, 167, 206
syphilis, 121
systemic model of symptom formation, 98
Szasz, Thomas, 28–30, 39, 44, 46

T

taxonomies, 119
technique de dépaysement, 183, 184
technology alibi, 108, 115
Temerlin, Maurice, 16, 39, 68, 182
test-retest reliability, 55, 59, 114
thick descriptions, 202, 204

thinking errors, 174
transferability, 200, 202, 204
transparency, 43, 92n4, 197
triangular model of symptom formation, 4, 100, 101, 116, 118, 162, 168
triangulation, 198, 199, 201, 203
trustworthiness, 180
truth-claims, 38, 39

U

unconscious, 15, 29, 92n4, 138, 171, 185
usability, 200, 201
US National Committee for Mental Hygiene, 12

V

validity
external, 200, 202, 204
internal, 200, 202–4
Van Os, Jim, 33, 47, 63, 91, 92, 110, 171, 206
Verhaeghe, Paul, 82, 92, 97, 103, 121, 140, 187
verification, 178, 193–7, 199
Verstehen, 5, 158–61
veterans, 13

W

Wakefield, Jerome, 155
Washington University, 15, 45
Westen, Drew, 28, 86
Western illness concept, 83
Whewell, William, 120

Whodas 2.0, 145
Why I Do Not Attend Case Conferences, 18, 69
Williams, Janet, 55–7, 55n12, 61, 63, 64
Winokur, George, 45
Woodruff, R.A., 48, 50
work discussions, 191–3, 192n6, 196, 197, 199, 203

World Health Organization (WHO), 1, 15, 145, 156, 157
World War II, 13
Wundt, Wilhelm, 176, 178

Z

Zachar, Peter, 122
Zanarini, M.C., 59

CPI Antony Rowe
Chippenham, UK
2017-08-21 22:37